Freeing the Butterfly

Transform Your Life Through Simple Exercises, Meditations, and Affirmations

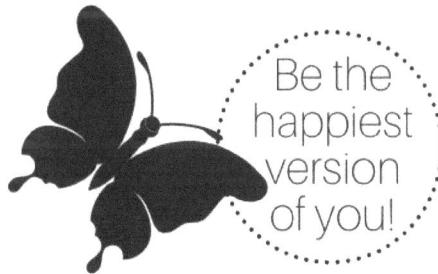

Be the happiest version of you!

Josie Myers

Michelle Cornish

Published by SolVin Creative.

ISBN 978-1-7750836-8-9

For Luca.

—J. M.

For anyone who's ever felt stuck. I hope this book brings you happiness.

—M. C.

Disclaimer

The authors of this book are not medical practitioners and as such, this book is not intended as a substitute for the medical advice of physicians or other practitioners. The reader should regularly consult a physician in matters relating to his/her health and particularly with respect to any symptoms that may require diagnosis or medical attention.

Acknowledgments

A special thanks to our beta readers, Kris and Lisa.

To our many spiritual teachers: We are grateful for your wisdom and guidance.

To Dr. Athena Perrakis for graciously agreeing to write a foreword for us.
Thank you for your support.

Contents

Foreword

Our planet is in a state of rapid flux and evolution, in case you haven't noticed, and so it brings me great personal and spiritual pleasure to see new books arriving onto the cosmic scene with real and actionable guidance to help support both where we are now and where we are heading to within the foreseeable future. Together, Josie and Michelle have united forces and frequencies to share their experiences and sacred wisdom; the result is a book full of practical wisdom and application that can, I believe, help prepare the reader to embody the energy needed for the coming times.

Throughout history we have considered ancient practices and peoples to be simplistic and underprepared for the times in which we live. And yet, more than ever I am seeing a resurgence of trust in ancient wisdom. In working with the seven chakra system here, the authors conjure the wisdom of the Vedas - the oldest recorded spiritual wisdom on this planet. By exploring the chakras in great detail, the authors create a physical roadmap to help the reader shift his or her current reality. Both women are so courageously confident and excited about their own healing, and through their words you get a sense of the long roads they themselves have traveled in order to arrive at their current state of healing. And while their stories are different, and of course different from yours, I have no doubt that you as reader will find yourself here. We are all one, and our healing looks both different and cosmically similar. There is one large road to Truth. On that road our journeys can look different but if you look closer and without a cynical eye, you can see how similarly Truth resonates across cultures, experiences, and identities.

What I love most about this book, and what I have found most enjoyable about it in my reading of it, is the way the authors incorporate playful exercises and inspiring journal prompts. As a writer myself, I process energetic experiences through language. If you are an artist who paints with color, or with oils, you will find the drawing space and invitation to bring your artistic skills to bear with an open heart. If you seek to embody your process more fully, each chapter includes yoga poses that incorporate chakra wisdom and sacred practice. Everything here is incredibly deep and rich, but offered in such a delicate and open way that anyone at any level of awareness will find the wisdom comforting, applicable, intoxicating, and uniquely personal.

May your process be fluid and full of beauty. I see the divine in you, and the authors do, too.

—**Athena Perrakis, Ph.D.**
Founder and CEO, Sage Goddess

What Does it Mean to 'Free the Butterfly'?

Have you ever wondered how a butterfly must feel to come out of its cocoon to a brand new world where it can fly and soar high into the sky? It's like they're a new and improved version of their old self, and we imagine it must feel pretty darn good.

That's what freeing the butterfly is all about—coming out of your funk, your cocoon, if you will, and feeling amazing with who you are.

When you read Josie and Michelle's stories, you will see they both went through this funk, and they noticed a lot of women around them going through similar experiences. It seems like when we're young, we try so hard to meet the expectations of people around us—parents, teachers, friends—that we forget about ourselves and what we want.

After a certain point, we realize doing all these things for other people does nothing for our own happiness. Many times something life-changing will happen to help us realize this, such as infertility, loss of a career, a serious accident, or the death of someone close to us. For other women, there's no major life event to trigger this transformation, they just realize they can't continue being unhappy, and it's time to find their spark again—time to wake up.

It's okay to feel uneasy at the mention of the word "spiritual" or the thought of having a "spiritual awakening". There's nothing to fear. Becoming more spiritual is simply being more conscious of what you need to feel happy, to love yourself, and be content with who you are—the real you. Often when we've lived a life of pleasing others, we really have no idea what we want for ourselves and what will make us happy. The tools in this book will help you discover that.

Through listening to other women and, in Josie's case, working with them in her energy practice, Josie and Michelle noticed several common stages that women who were awakening to their own desires experienced. In this book, we will walk you through each stage and give you some tools and strategies to get you to the next level and eventually to the point where you are maintaining that amazing feeling of soaring high in the sky like a beautiful butterfly.

We can't wait to guide you on this journey and help you free your inner butterfly.

About the Authors

Josie's Story

It was 2016, and I had been trying for three years to conceive my second child. I had difficulty conceiving my first child and was feeling the familiar strains of infertility creeping up on me: depression, anxiety, repressed feelings. I did not want to go down that road again. Infertility almost killed me. If you've ever experienced it, you know it affects you: body, mind, and soul.

My son played a huge part in helping me overcome my depression. I realized I needed to be there for him. While I wasn't going to be able to have a second child, I was damn sure I was going to be the best mom possible to my son.

Battling depression wasn't as easy as simply deciding I wasn't going to be depressed anymore. I was in a very dark place. When I asked my doctor for help, he quickly whipped out the prescription pad, but I refused. I wasn't interested in taking medication. While this works wonders for many people who suffer from depression, I knew it wasn't the right thing for me.

The thought of pouring my heart out to some stranger didn't appeal to me either. I wasn't interested in reliving past traumatic experiences and leaving the therapist's office a blubbering mess. That didn't feel right. And taking meds for depression felt like putting a bandaid on a wound to me.

I listened to my intuition. It was telling me there was more I needed to work on, and there was a way to do it without bringing up old emotional hurts. I just knew there had to be other options available. That's when I discovered energy healing.

I went for some Reiki sessions and started learning about chakras, spinning wheels of energy in our bodies. When chakras are blocked, this can cause physical, emotional, and mental symptoms like chronic bronchitis, moodiness, headaches, and depression. Once I learned how to clear, open, and keep my chakras functioning at their best, I started to feel so much better.

The difference was truly transformational.

It's important to listen to our intuition. If you feel something in the back of your mind or your gut telling you something's not right, listen. You're feeling that way for a reason. The voices in your head do serve a purpose.

I'm thankful I discovered the power of chakra healing, meditation, and affirmations, and I'm excited to share this information with you here in this book.

Michelle's Story

On the outside, I seemed to have it all: good health, a family who loved me, and a successful accounting practice. But inside I felt empty. For years I had been feeling like there was something more out there, like I was meant to do more with my life. The most exciting part of many of my days was getting the mail. I hoped there'd be something exciting in the mailbox, a sign from the universe to tell me how to get my mojo back. Crazy, right?

When my oldest son started kindergarten, I realized I wouldn't be able to pick him up from school because I needed to be at the office, and it broke my heart. I was torn between my clients and my family which was really no choice at all. Of course, my family won. I started taking the necessary steps to sell my accounting practice, and by the end of 2016 I was officially a stay-at-home mom.

I thought all my feelings of emptiness would magically disappear now that I had all the time in the world to spend with my family, but they didn't. The familiar feelings of stress and anxiety were still there. Now, I had new things to be stressed about. I felt like I had no purpose in life and my finances were a mess.

I had simply substituted one focus, my business, with another, my family. I still didn't know who I was or what I wanted. I connected with some friends online—my co-author, Josie, was one of them. She was the first person to teach me in-depth about the chakras and how they help us heal. My eyes were opened to a whole new way of thinking about how to create happiness. I learned about energy work and spiritual guidance and became more aware of who I wanted to be.

Most of all, I learned that happiness comes from within. I reconnected with activities I hadn't done for nearly twenty years, because I had lost the desire to do anything that wasn't going to advance my career or make me money.

The biggest thing this spiritual awakening taught me was that not only is it okay to do things just because they're fun, but it's also completely necessary for my wellbeing. That's a lesson I'm happy to share with my kids, and I'm looking forward to sharing it with you too.

The Tools Used in This Book

Each chapter in this book will guide you through a different stage in the process of freeing your inner butterfly and becoming a much happier version of yourself. You will find a number of tools to help you do this, each one tailored to the specific stage you are working through, to help you receive the most benefit from the work you are doing.

Below, you will find an introduction to the tools we will be working with. In each chapter, you are welcome to use all the tools, or pick and choose the ones that feel the most aligned with your healing process.

Energy Healing with the Chakras

Chakras are energy centers in the body. You can visualize them like small spinning discs inside your body. Chakra is a Sanskrit word meaning wheel or disc. When the chakras are unbalanced, they don't function properly, causing energy to get blocked in your body which causes symptoms exactly like what we were dealing with: stress, anxiety, depression, and a general sense we weren't living our best lives.

This doesn't even begin to cover the physical symptoms you can experience when your chakras are out of alignment! Physical symptoms can range from fatigue, headaches, and nausea to constipation, back aches, and sore throats.

There are seven chakras in all. Here's a quick rundown of each one, their Sanskrit name, and the symptoms you might experience if they aren't functioning at their best.

Root Chakra (Muladhara)

The root chakra is located at the bottom of your spine where your tailbone is and is represented by the color red. Because the root chakra is related to safety and security, when our basic survival needs aren't being met, the root chakra can become blocked.

Physical symptoms of a blocked root chakra can include low back pain, constipation, urinary issues, and knee and foot issues. Emotional symptoms of a blocked root chakra include codependency, financial worries, lack of focus, and not feeling secure in life.

Sacral Chakra (Svadhisthana)

The sacral chakra is located approximately two inches below the belly button. It is represented by the color orange and is related to creativity, pleasure, relationships, and sexual desire.

When the sacral chakra is blocked, you are likely to feel uninspired and have a low sex drive. Other emotional symptoms can include feeling unloved and unimportant. Physical symptoms of a blocked sacral chakra include abdominal cramping and changes in menstruation.

Solar Plexus Chakra (Manipura)

From the center of the belly button up to the breastbone is where you can find the solar plexus chakra. It is represented by the color yellow. The solar plexus is the core of your personal power and when it is blocked, you may be quick to anger or have digestive issues.

You may experience physical symptoms such as ulcers, gallstones, weight problems, or acid reflux. Emotionally, you may feel anxious or depressed and have a hard time with self-control and setting boundaries.

Heart Chakra (Anahata)

The heart chakra is located over your heart and is responsible for self love as well as love for others. When it isn't functioning properly, you may experience a loss of personal boundaries and feel unable to forgive others or yourself. It is represented by the color green.

Physical symptoms of a blocked heart chakra include heartburn, shoulder pain, difficulty breathing, and tightness in the chest.

Throat Chakra (Vishuddha)
When the throat chakra (located in the center of your collar bone, over your thyroid) isn't functioning properly, we have trouble speaking our truth with clarity. This can result in physical symptoms of a sore throat or cough. The color we associate with the throat chakra is light blue.

Third Eye Chakra (Ajna)
The third eye chakra is located between the eyebrows and is responsible for sensory perception, intuition, and psychic energy. Its color is indigo. Symptoms of a blocked third eye chakra include allergies, headaches, and a feeling of disconnection from spiritual experiences.

Crown Chakra (Sahasrara)
When the crown chakra is unbalanced, it is difficult for you to experience happiness, wisdom, and overall good health. Physical symptoms of a blocked crown chakra include poor memory, fatigue, headaches, and poor vision.

Among the emotional symptoms you might experience with a blocked crown chakra are isolation, depression, and the inability to make decisions. The crown chakra is located at the top of your head and is your connection to universal energy. It is associated with violet.

How Chakras Help You Heal
When the chakras aren't balanced, they don't function properly and you will experience a number of physical, emotional, and mental symptoms like what Josie experienced while dealing with infertility and Michelle experienced while feeling stressed and stuck.

The good news is, there are a number of simple things you can do to help balance and clear your chakras and you'll be learning about many of them in this book.

Yoga

We're sure you've heard about yoga. It's a great form of exercise but did you know it can help you stay grounded by keeping your chakras functioning optimally? It's also a great way to meditate if you have trouble sitting still. One of Josie's favorite ways to keep her chakras clear and balanced is using Mary Horsley's *Chakra Workout* book from the recommended resources section.

Throughout this book, you will find simple yoga poses to help with each chakra and transformation stage. If you want a more in-depth chakra yoga experience, we highly recommend Mary's book.

Affirmations

Affirmations are positive statements that affect the conscious and subconscious mind. They are usually short sentences, and you can say them out loud or to yourself. If you're not used to using affirmations, you may want to write them down and put them where you can see them, so you are reminded to say them often. The key is to say (or read) them many times throughout the day to continually reinforce the positive message contained within the affirmation.

Meditation

We both resisted meditation when it was first presented to us. We didn't want to sit cross-legged, chanting with our eyes closed. The good news is that's not what meditation is all about. There are many ways to meditate. Going for a walk outside is a great form of meditation!

The meditations in this book are meant to be visualization exercises to help you quickly escape the stresses of day-to-day life. If the idea of meditating overwhelms you, we've included coloring and doodling as alternatives.

Doodling & Coloring

Doodling and coloring are also great ways to meditate. Focusing on a blank page or a design you are coloring puts your brain in a relaxed state. We like the idea of doodling or coloring because you get the best of both worlds: a blank page and a pre-drawn image to color.

Some people are stressed by the thought of having to fill a blank page with doodles. The truth is, doodling is really just letting your mind wander and scribbling down whatever you think of. You can draw hearts or bubbles (or maybe butterflies?) over and over if that's what you feel like drawing. If this feels overwhelming, try coloring one of our pre-drawn images instead.

If the thought of coloring a whole page makes you anxious, then just color part of it or stick to the blank doodle pages. We've included both doodle and coloring pages in our book so you can choose what works best for you. Have fun and mix it up!

Markers (especially sharpies) will bleed through the page. If you plan to use them in this book, make sure you insert a piece of cardboard or some scrap pieces of paper under the page you are coloring to protect the other pages in the book.

Crystals

The healing benefits of crystals and stones are extraordinary. They are easy to use and you can find a crystal to help with almost anything you are dealing with. To use crystals, hold them in your hand while meditating, wear them (either as jewelry or in your pocket or bra), place them in your rooms, or put them in your purse.

Some types of crystals can also be used in bath or drinking water but be sure to check with your local crystal shop first to ensure this is safe both for you and the crystal (some will dissolve in water). Some crystals will fade when exposed to sunlight so you might want to ask about that as well.

There is one crystal that can be programmed. This means you can use it for anything, as long as you set your intentions, and tell the crystal what you want it to do. This is clear quartz. So, if you don't want to purchase all our recommended crystals but still want to try working with them, clear quartz is a great place to start.

Essential Oils

Known for their healing benefits, essential oils are the essences of plants, extracted in their purest form. There are varying qualities and grades of essential oils so make sure you are getting yours from a reputable source. The price can sometimes indicate the quality of the oil.

Inhaling the fragrances released from essential oils, allows the scent to stimulate your limbic system, the part of the brain contributing to emotions, behavior, sense of smell, and long-term memory.

In this book, we will focus on diffusing essential oils to take advantage of their benefits, but you can also apply them topically when diluted appropriately and take them orally as recommended. If you're not sure what the oil you have can be used for, always check the instructions on the bottle or ask an essential oil expert.

Journaling

Developing a routine journaling practice is the key to letting go of the stuff you don't need anymore so you can make room for new ideas and fresh perspectives. When Michelle first started journaling, she was reluctant to embrace the process and didn't believe the act of simply writing something down could help her deal with it and move on, but it did. The key to sticking with a journal practice is figuring out what works best for you.

You don't have to write pages and pages in your journal in order to start feeling better. In fact, you don't have to write at all. Sometimes sketching your thoughts works just as good, if not better than writing them in a journal. Michelle discovered that a combination of the two works best for her. Sometimes she prefers to draw about her day and other times she likes to write. Sometimes she writes bullet points, and sometimes she writes poetry.

The reason journaling works to help you start healing and feeling better, is that it gets your thoughts out of your head and onto paper. There are two types of journaling practices we recommend you try to make a daily habit: gratitude and releasing.

Gratitude
A gratitude journal is where you list all the things you are thankful for every day. If you've had a bad day, this can be difficult. A gratitude journal helps remind us to be thankful for even the most basic things like taking a breath and drinking clean water. The more you find to feel grateful for, the more you will find your day wasn't as bad as you thought it was.

Releasing
We highly recommend you keep a separate journal for releasing negativity. This could even be a piece of loose paper that isn't in a journal, because you may want to burn it or rip it up afterwards. This can be very freeing.

The purpose of releasing is to help you let go of negative thoughts and energy. In your releasing journal, you will write all the negative things you think about. These are things like not feeling good enough, not liking the way you look, not loving yourself, etc. Don't edit yourself. Just write until you feel like all those negative thoughts are out of your head and on the paper.

After you've finished writing down all your negative thoughts, destroy the paper (safely, of course). As you are ripping up, burning, shredding, or flushing those tiny bits of paper, think about letting all those thoughts go and giving them to the universe to take care of for you. You no longer need to burden yourself with these kinds of thoughts.

1

Recognizing You're Stuck

"Growth is painful. Change is painful. But nothing is as painful as staying stuck somewhere you don't belong."

—*Mandy Hale*

Recognizing you're stuck can be one of the most difficult things to do because it's a sign that you need help. Many people see needing help as a sign of weakness, but it's actually quite the opposite. By taking action and reading this book, you are making a commitment to yourself to live a happier life. You are telling yourself you are valuable and you are strong.

It's okay to feel stuck. All butterflies must first be caterpillars, stuck on the ground, before they can spread their wings and fly. The important thing is that you recognize you are stuck and you're willing to investigate ways of getting unstuck.

When you are stuck in your life, you may experience a range of different emotions from feeling angry and triggered to not feeling much of anything at all, like you're numb. It's common to feel very alone and even abandoned when you're stuck. A stuck person typically looks to other people to find happiness rather than discovering their own joy from within. It feels a bit like you've lost control of your own life.

Chakras

When you're stuck, your root and solar plexus chakras aren't balanced. Remember, the root chakra is located at the base of your spine and is responsible for your safety, security, and self-preservation. Symptoms of not feeling safe and secure include feelings of abandonment, loneliness, and sadness. Physical symptoms of an unbalanced root chakra include lower back pain, constipation, diarrhea, and problems with the groin, hips, or legs.

The solar plexus chakra is all about personal power and self-esteem. When we look to other people to make us happy and we have low self-esteem, our solar plexus chakra is out of balance. An unbalanced solar plexus chakra can cause physical symptoms such as constipation, binge eating, acid reflux, weight issues, and even addiction.

Yoga Pose

The root chakra helps us feel grounded, so when it's out of balance, we lack a sense of objectivity and the ability to see things the way they really are. When we're grounded we feel more balanced and sensible.

The yoga pose we've chosen to help you feel more grounded and start getting unstuck is the thunderbolt pose. To get in the thunderbolt position, sit on your yoga mat in a kneeling position, legs hip-width apart, buttocks on your heels. Rest your hands comfortably on your thighs and lengthen the back of your neck by tucking in your chin.

Close your eyes or gaze at the floor, looking about three feet in front of you. Take a few deep breaths. Rest in this pose for as long as you need to. Concentrate on visualizing a connection to the earth and feeling safe and supported. The thunderbolt pose promotes security and peacefulness and improves posture and aligns your spine.

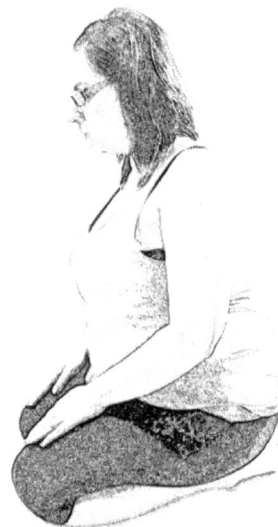

Affirmations

If you've never used affirmations before, it may feel a little weird saying them out loud at first. That's totally normal. You can say them to yourself if that feels more comfortable.

- · I feel safe and secure.
- · I create my own happiness.
- · I am ready to feel happy.

Make a conscious effort to repeat these affirmations several times throughout the day. If your day is hectic, here are a few tips to help you get your affirmations in:

- Say the affirmations before getting out of bed in the morning,
- Set an alarm to remind yourself to say the affirmations,
- Set a timer for five minutes and repeat the affirmations until the time is up,
- Write the affirmations on sticky notes and post them on your mirror or somewhere else you will see them regularly, or
- Write the affirmations over and over in your journal.

Meditation

Sit in a comfortable position with your feet on the floor. Close your eyes and take three slow, deep breaths. Imagine your feet are growing roots and the roots are extending far into the center of the earth. Now imagine a read ball of light floating up to your root chakra. When it gets there, the light expands to surround you.

Soak in the light for as long as you like. Now imagine the light entering your root chakra. Repeat the affirmation, "I am safe," and feel the glowing red light filling your body with energy. The energy is there for you whenever you need it. Visualize the light shrinking into your root chakra. Be still and notice what comes to you. Simply observe. Don't worry about trying to make sense of your thoughts. Let them come and go freely.

When you're ready, take a deep breath and open your eyes. You may feel like you need a drink of water or you may want to have your journal handy to take some notes about your experience. You should feel relaxed and calmer than before the meditation.

As an alternative to the visual meditation, you can color or doodle on the following pages.

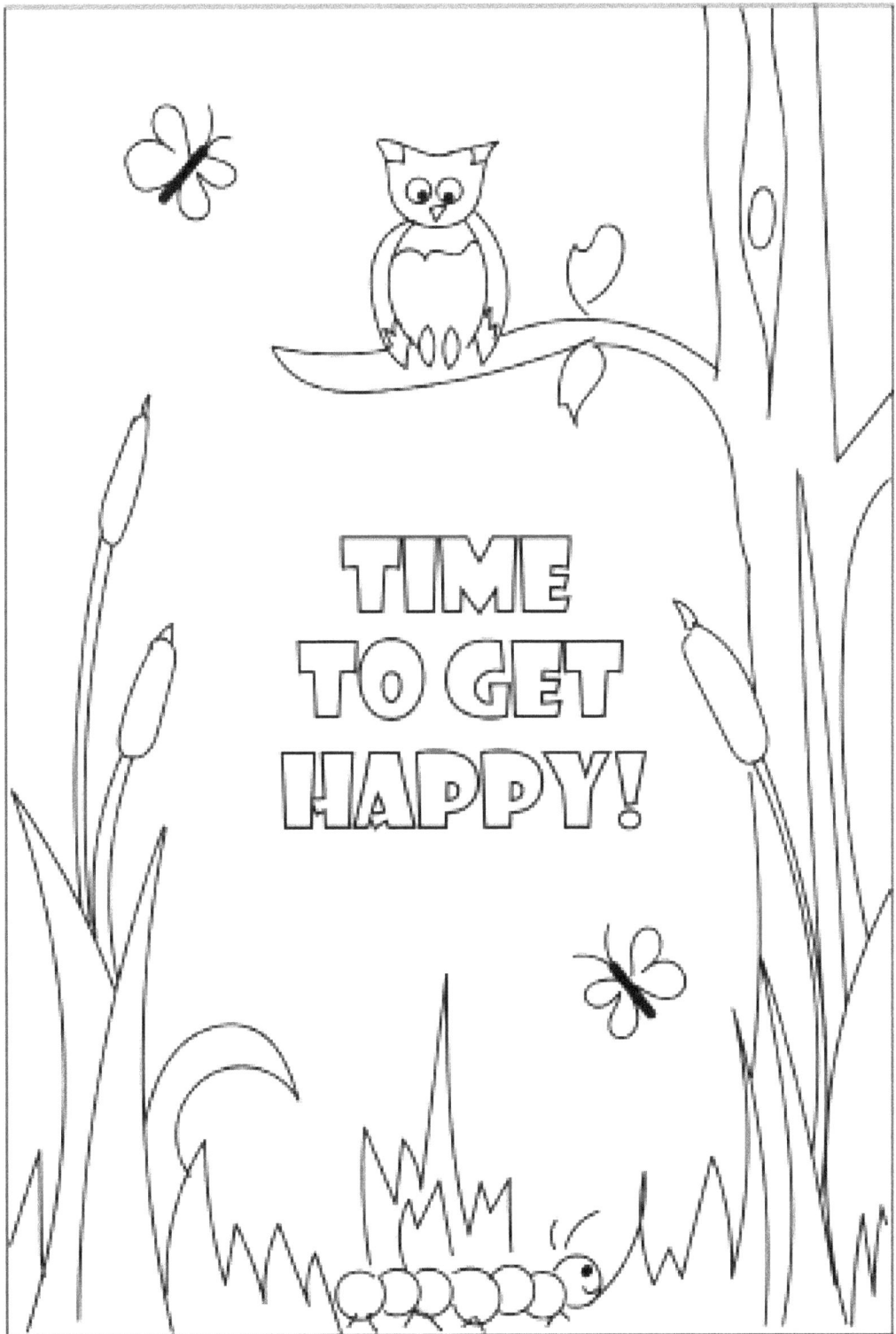

TIME
TO GET
HAPPY!

Use this page to **DOODLE**. If using markers, you may want to place extra paper or a piece of cardboard under this page to prevent bleed through. Have fun!

Crystals

Bloodstone is a great crystal to support the root chakra. You can hold it in your hand while you meditate, place it on your bedside table while you sleep, or just have it somewhere near you. Because bloodstone supports the root chakra you might also try putting it in a pocket that is near your root chakra for maximum benefits.

This crystal is dark green with dark red spots resembling spots of blood which is where it gets its name. Bloodstone is great for grounding (connecting to the earth) and works to remove negative energy from the body.

To support your solar plexus and encourage feelings of personal power and high self-esteem, we recommend working with citrine. Citrine is from the quartz family and is a beautiful yellow. Citrine is one of the crystals that is safe to use in the bath, so if you enjoy taking baths, try putting it in your bath and see how you feel.

You can also use citrine in the same ways mentioned for bloodstone. Remember, your solar plexus chakra is located midway between the breast bone and the belly button so wearing it in your bra or as a necklace will provide great support for your solar plexus chakra.

Most crystals can be purchased inexpensively as a small stone, however, as mentioned in the introduction, if you don't want to buy a lot of crystals, you can use clear quartz instead of any of the crystals we recommend.

To use clear quartz instead of any other crystal, you must tell the clear quartz how you want it to help you. This is called programming your crystal. You can do this in your mind by visualizing what you want the crystal to do. We know if you're not used to working with crystals, it can seem a bit silly to talk out loud to your crystal, but it really works!

We recommend telling all your crystals what you want help with and asking them to guide you.

Essential Oils

Because the root chakra is closest to the earth, any earthy oil will be a great support. Frankincense is one we recommend. It comes from the Boswellia tree and has many healing properties like fighting inflammation, boosting immune system function, preventing signs of aging, and reducing stress and negative emotions. We recommend diffusing frankincense or diluting it with a carrier oil like coconut oil and rubbing it on your wrists. You can also try rubbing the diluted mixture on your hips to get closer to your root chakra.

Some oils to try for supporting the solar plexus are ginger and anything citrus. Ginger and citrus can both burn when used on the skin (even when diluted) so we recommend diffusing this oil. If you don't have a diffuser, you can put a drop of oil on a cotton ball or mix a spray bottle with oil and water or rubbing alcohol.

Journal Prompt

For your releasing journal, write about the negative feelings you are experiencing the most right now. In this stage of feeling stuck, you are likely feeling abandoned, lonely, sad, angry, or just plain irritated. It's also common to not really know what you're feeling. That's the numbness talking. It's okay to write about not knowing how you feel or even just the first thing that comes to mind.

On the following page or in a separate journal, answer the question: How am I feeling about my life right now?

In your gratitude journal or on the following page, remember to write down at least ten things you are thankful for today. If you want, you can focus on things that make you feel safe like nourishing food, a roof over your head, clean water to drink, etc. There are always things to be grateful for.

Summary

It's okay to feel stuck. In fact, if you're feeling stuck in your life, you should congratulate yourself for recognizing this. In this chapter, you learned that feeling stuck results in loneliness, abandonment, and loss of control over your own life.

When the root chakra and solar plexus chakra aren't balanced, they can contribute to feeling stuck. Practice the thunderbolt pose and feeling connected to the earth. Remember that you create your own happiness. Working with crystals like bloodstone and citrine and using essential oils like frankincense and ginger can help your chakras while you get unstuck.

Action Step

Choose at least three of the tools above and use them every day. Bonus points if you use *all* the tools every day!

Celebrate that you have recognized you are stuck and have taken the first step toward your healing. Do something nice for yourself that you enjoy. This can be something simple like indulging in a fancy coffee, taking a relaxing bath, or buying a new notebook.

2

Committing to Making a Change

"It's far better to live your own path imperfectly than to live another's path perfectly."

—*Bhagavad Gita*

Let's face it—change is hard. If it was easy, we would do it all the time and everyone would be walking around in a permanent state of bliss. You often know in your gut when it's time to make a change. You might receive some signals, see some signs, or feel that your intuition is telling you it's time.

When you're ready to commit to making a change, you may feel a bit angry with yourself. It's like you're putting your foot down and telling yourself you're tired of how things have been, and it's time to do something about it. You might feel like you're at your wit's end and just don't know what else to do other than change. Maybe you're simply tired of how things have been.

Whatever you're feeling, you know it's time to do something about it and you're ready to do this for yourself. To revisit the butterfly metaphor, think about the caterpillar getting ready to make a cocoon. Here she's finding a good spot to hunker down and focus on herself for a while. That's what you'll be doing too. It's time to commit to making a change so you can emerge from your cocoon in a more blissful state.

Chakras

Once again, we are going to be focusing on your root and solar plexus chakras. When you're ready to make a commitment to change, you need to feel like it's safe to do so and that's your root chakra talking. We're going to work on clearing and balancing the root chakra so you are more comfortable and less scared with the process of change. You need to change so you can preserve yourself, and focusing on your root chakra will help you do that.

The solar plexus chakra, the one responsible for personal power, is going to help during this stage by making sure you can muster the strength needed to make this commitment to yourself. Self-mastery is required when we make a big change like this, and focusing on balancing and healing your solar plexus chakra will help you discover what it is you really want during this process.

Yoga Pose

Tree Pose
Stand barefoot on a yoga mat or wherever you feel comfortable keeping your balance. Place your feet about hip distance apart with your hands at your side. Lift your right foot and place it on your left leg at the inner thigh, above the knee, or at the calf so that your right knee is pointing to the right side. Do not place your right foot at your left knee. You want to avoid any pressure on your joints.

You may need to use your right hand to help you position your leg and that is fine. Place your palms together at your heart. Play around with your gaze. Some people feel like they have better balance when they look at the floor and others find it easier to look straight ahead.

Hold for as long as feels comfortable to you and repeat one of the affirmations below or just relax and focus on your breathing. If you have good balance, you can try raising your gaze to look up and even lifting your arms towards the sky like the branches of a tree.

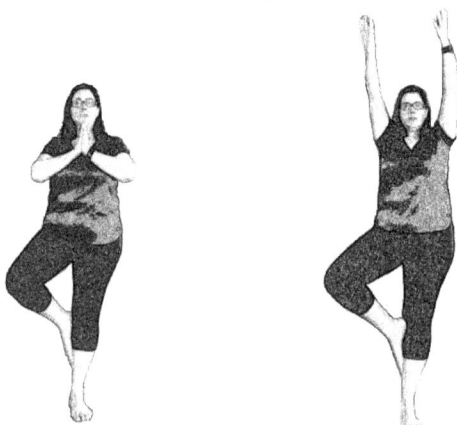

Affirmations

We want you to know that it is safe to change. If you choose to work with one affirmation from this chapter, choose:

· It's safe to change.

These affirmations are great variations of it's safe to change:

· I have the power to change.
· I have what it takes to make a change.
· I can flourish.

Make a conscious effort to repeat these affirmations several times throughout the day. If your day is hectic, refer to Chapter 1 for some ways to help you remember to repeat your affirmations. Here are a few more:

· Use the affirmation (or part of it) as your password,
· Make up a song using your affirmations that you can sing to yourself in the car while driving,
· Write the affirmations in lipstick on your mirror,
· Create some art using the affirmation,
· Write the affirmation (or choose one significant word) and doodle around it in your journal.

Meditation

Sit or lay down in a comfortable position. Close your eyes, take a deep breath in and slowly let it out. Imagine a white light surrounding and comforting you. Think about your future self and what your life will be like once you complete this transformation and are able to live a happy, fulfilled life. Sit with your thoughts for a few moments and notice what comes to you.

When you have a clear picture of what you want your life to be like, enjoy the moment. If you're having a hard time picturing yourself happy, that's okay. When we deny ourselves happiness, it can be difficult to remember what brings us joy. Just notice what thoughts come to you.

When you are ready, open your eyes. You may want to journal about what you saw to reinforce your visualization. What were you wearing? How did you look? How did you feel?

Just like in Chapter 1, you have the option of coloring or doodling instead of meditating. You'll find a spot for that next.

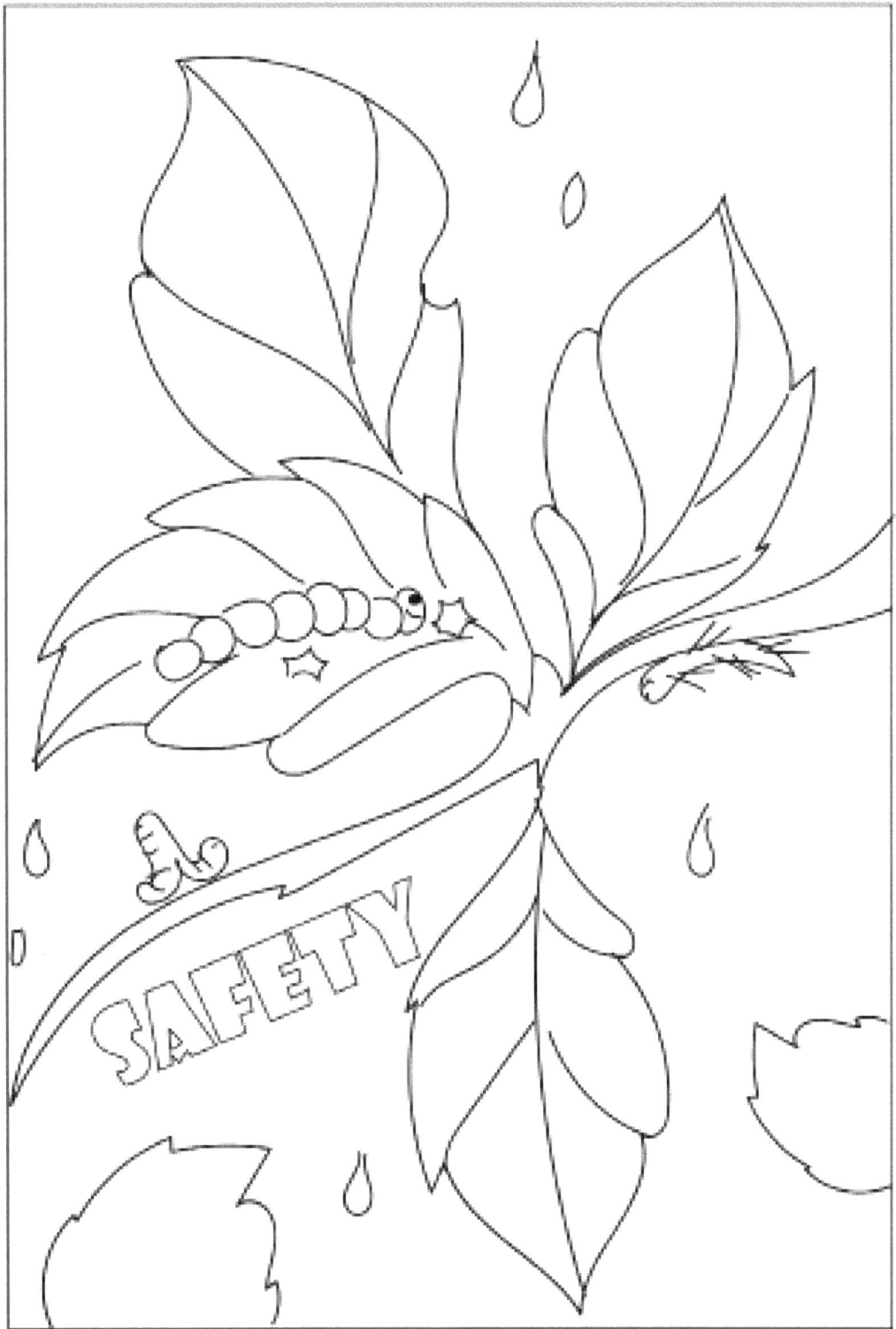

Use this page to **DOODLE**. If using markers, you may want to place extra paper or a piece of cardboard under this page to prevent bleed through. Have fun!

Crystals

Unakite is another wonderful crystal to support your root chakra. It is a pink and green stone from the granite family and is a popular stone for craft jewellery. As a combination of red jasper and epidote, unakite is the perfect stone to help release deep-seated emotions in a gentle way, allowing you to feel safe as you rid yourself of the unwanted emotions that are holding you back.

When you are in a state of feeling stuck and deciding to make a change, it is easy to feel overwhelmed. Unakite can help by reminding you to focus on the present moment. Use unakite by wearing it as jewellery, keeping it in your pocket or bra, or placing it around your house to remind you that you are safe to commit to making this change.

To support your solar plexus chakra, we recommend amber. Amber is a yellowish orange color and is fossilized resin produced by extinct coniferous trees. You are probably familiar with amber jewellery. Because amber helps to alleviate inflammation, amber necklaces are often used to help ease teething pain, as well as muscle pain and arthritis.

When it comes to the emotional benefits of amber, it helps to ease anxiety by reducing fatigue and helping you feel more open to new experiences. Amber is considered to be the most beneficial when it heats up, therefore, to receive the most benefit from amber, it's important that it touches your body as often as possible. This can include holding it in your hand while you go about your day, meditating with it in your hand, or putting it in your bra.

Essential Oils

In this chapter, we are continuing to focus on the root and solar plexus chakras. Lavender oil is great for the root chakra because it's very calming and can reduce any fears you have about making a commitment to yourself, helping you to feel safe. It helps to shift your awareness and perspective and has been shown to help with anxiety, depression, and restlessness.

Diffuse lavender when going to bed or dilute it with coconut oil and rub on the soles of your feet. An Epsom salt bath with lavender oil is also very relaxing. Mix a few drops of the oil with the Epsom salts before adding them to the bath water.

Bergamot essential oil also helps to alleviate feelings of depression, but in a slightly different way, because it helps to balance your solar plexus chakra, rather than you root chakra. Because it is a citrus oil, bergamot stimulates feelings of cheerfulness and helps to increase your energy.

This is a great oil to diffuse in the morning or throughout the day to give you a little boost. If you're not able to diffuse oils throughout the day, carry a bottle of bergamot essential oil with you to smell whenever you need a pick me up. Dilute with coconut oil and apply to wrists or behind your ears if you're comfortable using essential oils topically.

Journal Prompt

For this journal prompt, we want you to think about what scares you about making a big change in your life.

In your releasing journal, or on the next page, write about all the fears you have about becoming a different person. Whatever pops into your mind, write it down. Sometimes our thoughts don't make sense right away but as you write, you gain clarity. For example, sometimes we fear being happy. If something like this comes up for you then ask yourself why and write about it.

Remember, it's okay if you don't know what you are feeling right now. Simply write about that. A limiting belief is something we think about that keeps us feeling stuck and unhappy. It's important to get all those limiting beliefs out of your head so you can start thinking more clearly about what you truly desire.

Answer the question: What are my limiting beliefs about changing?

In your gratitude journal, remember to write down at least ten things you are thankful for today. If you remember a time when there was a change in your life that you were grateful for, write about that. Or, if you did the meditation, write about what you were grateful for seeing in your visualization.

Summary

Here, again, we've focused on the root and solar plexus chakras. These are the chakras that are going to help you commit to making a change and feel safe in doing so. To support the balancing and clearing of these chakras, you can try the yoga pose. We like doing tree pose while saying one or more of the affirmations.

Remember, you have the power to change and you are safe. Change is an important and necessary part of living a happy life. For more support, practice your preferred form of meditation, call on the power of unakite and amber, and use lavender and bergamot essential oils.

Action Step

Think about your happiness. What do you see for yourself? Is there something you can implement right now? If you visualized your future self, were you wearing something you already own or doing something you can do right now? Try drawing your vision of your happier and self.

3

Trying Something New

"Just try new things. Don't be afraid. Step out of your comfort zones and soar, all right?"

—*Michelle Obama*

So, you've committed to making a change. Now we're going to take that a step further and try some new things to get you used to stepping out of your comfort zone. Change isn't something that happens overnight and it isn't an easy process, but now that you've committed to the process, you might as well get used to trying new things. You might find you really enjoy some of them!

In order to change into a beautiful butterfly, a caterpillar must hang upside down so it can start to form its cocoon. Talk about stepping out of your comfort zone!

You will know you're in this stage of your transformation when you begin to notice things you weren't even aware of before. This can range from little things, like a new way of completing a daily task, all the way to big things like wanting to become vegan or go on a spiritual retreat. Look for things that will help you transition to a happier version of yourself.

What brings you joy?

The best way to discover this is to try many things and experiment as you go. You might want to make some notes in your journal so you'll know which things you are enjoying and which things you can do without. Keep a notebook or use the memo function on your phone so you can remember which things you want to try as you think of them.

Chakras

In this chapter, we will be focusing on your sacral and solar plexus chakras. The sacral chakra helps with creativity and self-expression, so it will help you come up with ideas for new things you'd like to try. When your sacral chakra is blocked, you might feel like you've lost control of your life, like you're walking around in a state of numbness.

When your sacral chakra isn't functioning at its best, you can experience physical symptoms like abdominal pain or changes in your menstrual cycle. You may feel unmotivated and have a low sex drive.

By trying new things and continuing to do the activities you enjoy, you are taking control of your life and your happiness. The solar plexus chakra will help you do that too. A time for trying new things is a time to step into your personal power and own your right to be happy by doing things you enjoy.

When your solar plexus is blocked, you can end up letting other people make all the decisions for you. This can sometimes result in you not feeling like you know what you want. That's okay. As you work through this chapter, you will start to rediscover yourself and really understand what you enjoy.

It's time to focus on you. You're in your cocoon figuring out what you really want in life.

Yoga Pose

Cobra Pose
Cobra pose is a great posture for realigning the spine and improving circulation to the pelvis.

Step 1: Lie on your stomach and relax, stretching out your legs. Place your forehead on the mat and your hands palms down with your arms bent and your hands under your shoulders.

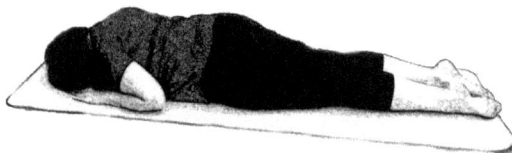

Step 2: Inhale and lengthen the back of your neck. Exhale and raise your forehead, nose, chin, shoulders, and upper back and chest in a snake like movement. Try and only use your arms for balance. Hold the pose and breath for a few moments. Visualize an orange light in your pelvis and say to yourself, "I open my creativity".

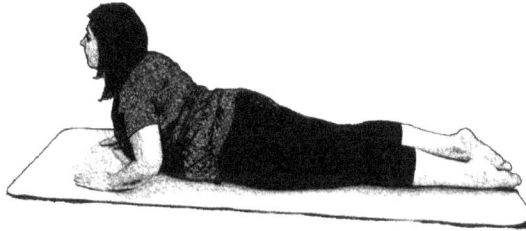

Step 3: Exhale while slowly uncurling your spine, lowering your chest, chin, and nose until your forehead rests on the mat. Repeat this pose three times.

Affirmations

The following affirmations will help you get the most out of this stage of your transformation.

· I welcome new experiences.
· I find excitement in new experiences.
· I express myself in new ways.

Since this chapter focuses on trying new things, see if you can come up with some new ways to use your affirmations. If you've been taping them to your mirror, try putting them near your coffee pot. Express your creativity and create a doodle or piece of art that uses one or more of the affirmations. Record voice memos of the affirmations to play for yourself whenever you need a pick me up.

Meditation

Think of something you've never tried before or something you haven't done in a number of years because you've been too nervous. Sit or lie in a comfortable position. Close your eyes and imagine yourself doing that activity you've been wanting to do.

See and feel how much joy it brings you. Can you see the smile on your face? Do you feel the lightness and excitement in your body while you take part in this activity? Are you alone or is someone with you? Take as long as you want to relax and feel all the happiness this activity brings you. When you are ready, take a deep breath and open your eyes.

Now make a plan to do the activity you just visualized. It can be a small step to start with. If you were singing on stage, maybe you want to practice in front of a small group of supportive friends first. Each small step in the direction of happiness counts.

The coloring and doodle pages are here for you to use too.

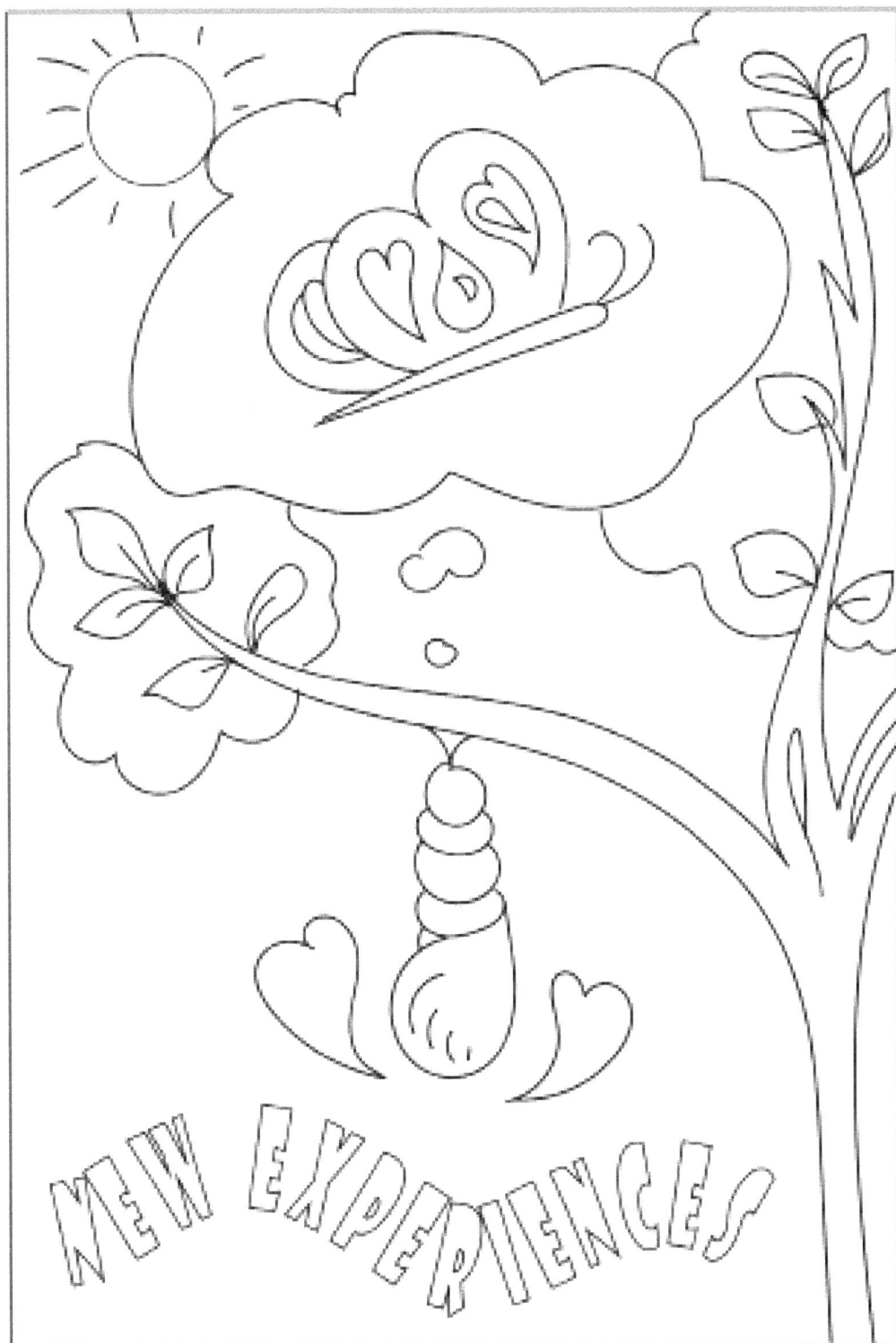

NEW EXPERIENCES

Use this page to **DOODLE**. If using markers, you may want to place extra paper or a piece of cardboard under this page to prevent bleed through. Have fun!

Crystals

The color associated with the sacral chakra is the orange. Carnelian is a semi-precious stone that comes in orange or orange-red varieties. The benefits of working with carnelian include increased confidence and creativity.

Carnelian is said to bring out your true self. To work with carnelian, you can wear jewellery made of the stone, carry a piece of carnelian in your purse, bra, or pocket, or put a piece on your desk or other work space.

A great crystal for amplifying personal power is tiger eye. This crystal helps open up and strengthen your solar plexus chakra. Tiger eye is a brownish crystal with bands of yellow-gold. It's great for releasing fear and allowing us to take action. You will also find that when you work with tiger eye, you have an easier time making decisions because you are able to look at your choices more objectively. Use it in the same way you use carnelian.

Try alternating how you use your crystals so you can see which methods work the best for you. You can also alternate which crystal you wear so you get a clear sense of how each crystal is affecting you.

Essential Oils

Ylang ylang essential oil is made from the flowers of the herb Cananga odorata genuina. It is very fragrant with a sweet fruity, floral scent. It can be used to support the sacral chakra by promoting relaxation and reducing blood pressure. It's also a great mood and energy booster. Diffuse or dilute and apply topically.

To support your solar plexus chakra during this stage of your transformation, we recommend cinnamon essential oil. The benefits of cinnamon essential oil include reducing stress and increasing energy. Cinnamon has a number of physical benefits too, like helping to prevent cancer and heart disease. For an extra boost, add cinnamon spice (not the essential oil) to any foods you like.

Cinnamon is a hot oil which means it can burn when applied to the skin. For this reason, you may want to avoid applying it topically.

Journal Prompt

Answer the following questions in your journal.

- · What have you wanted to try but haven't? Why not?
- · What are some experiences you've wanted to have but haven't? Why not?
- · Why is now a good time to try those things?

If you feel like now is not a good time to try new things, journal about that too. There are no wrong answers—just insights to help you on your journey. Remember, you can release any negative feelings by writing them in a journal or on a piece of paper then safely burning or shredding it.

In your gratitude journal, write about why you are thankful for the opportunity to try new things. Try to come up with ten reasons. If you get stuck, you can write about other things you are thankful for.

Summary

We're excited that you are starting to try new things and noticing things about yourself that you didn't before! Ensuring your sacral chakra and solar plexus chakra are functioning at their best will help you feel more confident as you continue to enjoy new experiences.

Remember to try the cobra pose and practice your affirmations. Expressing yourself in new ways can be scary but there is also something very empowering about being true to yourself and your desires. Continue to use the tools we recommend. If there are some you haven't tried yet, now is a great time to try a new one!

Action Step

Trying new things can be scary. Even if it's something small like trying a new flavor or brand of coffee, try something new every week. Work your way up to bigger things. You will find that when you start with little things, you will quickly gain the courage to try bigger things.

Remember to use your crystals and oils for support. In the next chapter, we will be discussing how to find supportive people to help you on your journey.

4

Finding Support

"Find someone who knows you're not perfect but treats you as if you are."

—Unknown

I know you've heard this before—change is hard! While a butterfly transforms in its cocoon, thanks to the magic of mother nature, it's much more difficult for us humans to make such amazing transformations, especially on our own. In the last chapter, you made a commitment to change for the sake of your happiness. This is a big step. Now, let's talk about how you can find some support to increase your chances of success.

You are much more likely to achieve your goals if you share them with someone, but it's important that it's not just anyone that you share them with. When going through a major life transformation, you want to seek out people who are going to support you no matter what. The last thing you want is for the person you are hoping will help you to end up taking off when things get tough.

It's also not helpful to have people telling you what *they* think you should do. This is usually based on their judgment of your actions and truly supportive people aren't judgmental, they want to see you succeed in a way that is best for you. So, how do you find these supportive people?

If you are experiencing any medical symptoms related to stress, anxiety, depression, and the like, you can start by consulting with your doctor. Ask them if they can recommend a professional counselor or some support groups you can visit. Many communities have free support groups that can be very helpful. Local community centers will have a list of local support groups as well.

It may take a few tries to find a group that feels right to you, and that's totally okay. If you don't feel comfortable, you won't feel supported. Try not to get discouraged if this happens to you. It may take some time to find the right support, but once you do, it will be worth it.

There are also many support groups online. You can find free forums and Facebook and LinkedIn groups related specifically to the types of things you are dealing with. We have found the spiritual community to be very supportive and non-judgmental. There are varying degrees of spirituality, so it may take you a few tries to find the group that feels like a good fit for you. Don't get discouraged, this is totally normal.

You may already have a very supportive friend or family member you can turn to for support, and that is perfect. When looking for support, you want to look for a person or group who is going to be around for the long haul. Unfortunately, it's not as simple as asking the person if they plan to stick around, so it may be hard to tell at first who is going to provide the best support for you. If you're considering joining a group, see if you can find out how long they have been active or how many members they have.

People come and go in our lives, and you may find this happens to you as you are going through this transformation. Sometimes the people that were good for us at one stage of our lives are no longer good for us later in our journey. It's not their fault and it's certainly not yours, it's just part of life. The important thing to remember is that you always have the ability to ask for help. Make sure you remember that. People don't always instinctively know if you need help, so you'll have to find the courage to ask for it. And if you find that someone who was once a great support to you is no longer there when you need them, recognize this, and find someone else you can talk to.

Chakras

The chakras that will help you ask for support are the root chakra and the throat chakra. Remember that the root chakra helps you feel safe and secure—grounded. When we feel safe, it's easier for us to ask for support. The throat chakra also comes into play here because we need to use our voice when asking for help, so having a balanced throat chakra will allow you to do this.

When we live our lives based on what is expected of us, rather than how we feel we should, both the root and throat chakras become unbalanced. The symptom most associated with an unbalanced root chakra, as it relates to asking for support, is a lack of confidence. When our root chakra is out of balance, we lack confidence and, in extreme situations, we can feel paranoid for no reason. You feel like your life is out of control.

Living our lives how we feel we should instead of how we want to also results in a blocked throat chakra which causes symptoms like struggling to verbalize our thoughts, feeling like we don't have a voice, participating in restrictive relationships, and manifesting physical issues such as sore throats, coughs, or thyroid problems.

Finding those people who are going to support you no matter what is going to go a long way to helping you live a happier life, but it can take courage to do so. The exercises in this chapter are designed to help you balance your root and throat chakras so you will feel more confident as you ask for help and find support on your journey to becoming the happiest version of you!

Yoga Pose

Chin Lock
The chin lock pose focuses energy on your throat chakra and helps release a stiff neck.

Step 1: Sit in a comfortable cross-legged post.

Step 2: Inhale then lower your head until your chin is pressed against your chest. Hold your breath for a few seconds, then exhale.

Step 3: When you are ready to inhale again, release the chin lock and lift your head back to an upright position.

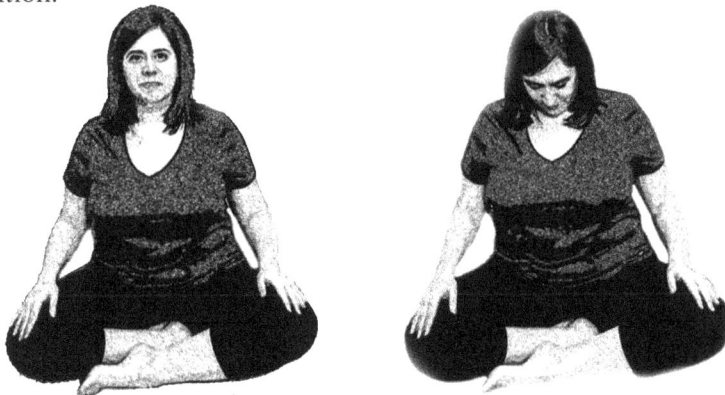

Affirmations

These affirmations will support you as you reach out for support and connect with people who can help you on your transformation journey.

· I am supported.
· I find support easily.
· I am connected.

By now you are starting to get quite the collection of affirmations you can use every day. Just because we are focusing on finding support in this chapter, doesn't mean you have to stop using affirmations from the previous chapters. These are just suggestions. If you find you are drawn to affirmations from the other chapters, then go ahead and use them.

Meditation

The goal of this chapter is to help you feel supported, so let's get you visualizing that perfect person or group of people who are going to support you in the happiest version of your life.

Find a comfortable spot to sit or lie down. Close your eyes and focus on your breath. Inhale and exhale, long and slow. Picture yourself as the happiest you've ever been. Try to see what you're wearing. It's okay if the details aren't clear to you. If you have a favorite outfit, imagine yourself wearing it.

Is there anyone in your vision with you? Do you already know them or is it someone you've never met before? See if you can picture them. See their face. Their kind eyes and gentle smile are comforting. Sit with your vision as long as you like, imagining who will come into your life to support you while you become a happier version of yourself.

When you're ready, open your eyes and take a deep breath. Say thank you to the people who showed up in your vision to support you, even if you don't know who they are yet. You are loved and supported. Now flip to a page in your journal, or use the journal page provided in this chapter, to write about who you saw and how it felt having them support you.

Remember, you can always color or doodle if you don't feel like visualizing or meditating today.

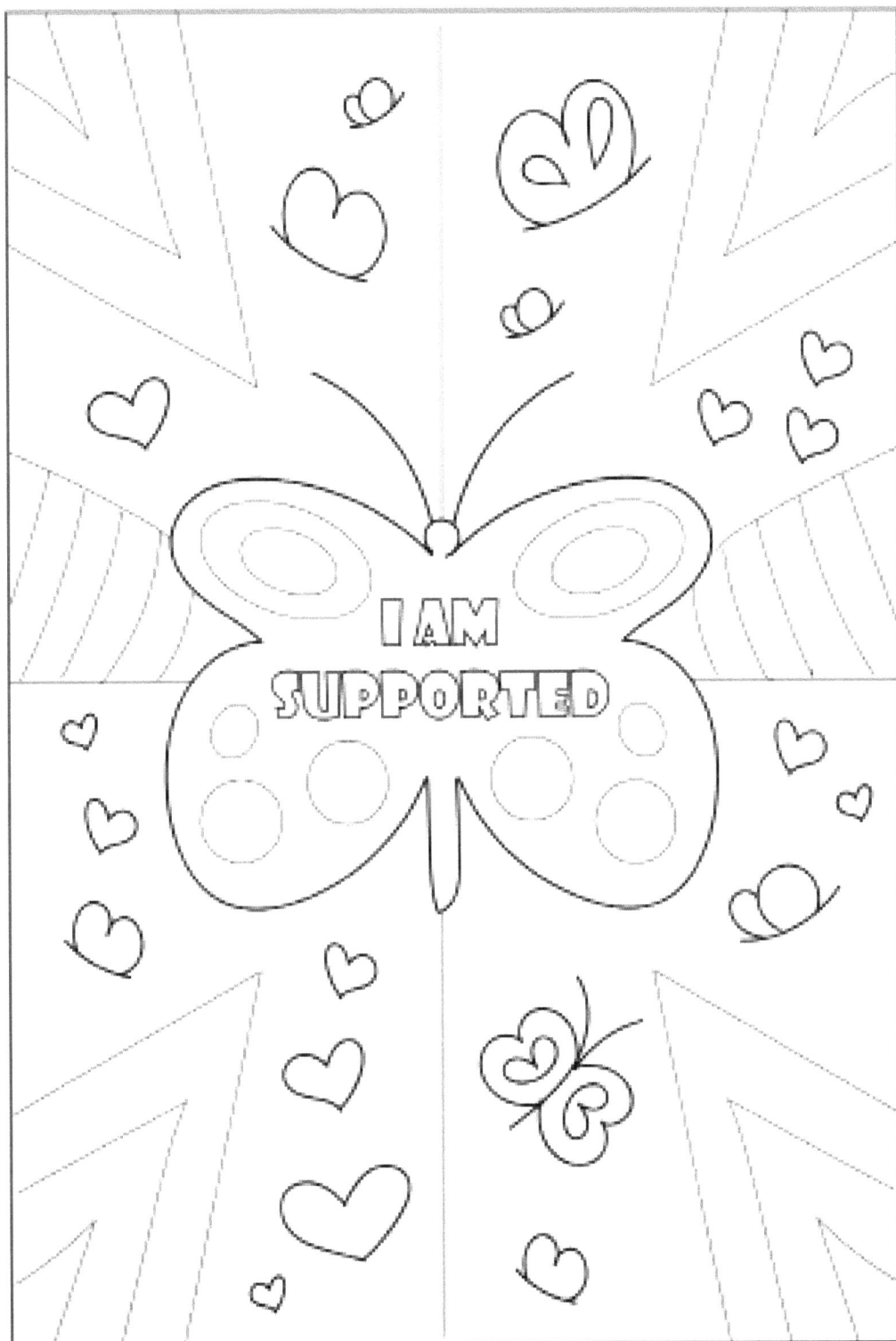

I AM SUPPORTED

Use this page to **DOODLE**. If using markers, you may want to place extra paper or a piece of cardboard under this page to prevent bleed through. Have fun!

Crystals

We have already discussed two wonderful crystals you can use to support your root chakra: bloodstone and unakite. If you have these crystals, go ahead and use them. Another wonderful crystal to use with your root chakra is obsidian.

Obsidian protects you from fear, anxiety, and anger and is often known as the psychic cleanser because it's so good at removing bad vibes. Its formed from molten lava that has cooled so quickly it didn't have time to turn into glass, and, because it is found all over the world, it's often easy to come by. It's quite common to find jewellery made of obsidian.

A great crystal to use when working with the throat chakra is blue lace agate. Blue lace agate is a light sky-blue color with striations of slightly lighter and darker blue that form a banded appearance. Blue lace agate is a stone of encouragement and support and can assist with communication, so if you feel like you need a little help asking for support, then blue lace agate is your stone.

Use your obsidian or blue lace agate in the way you find most comfortable: placing it somewhere in your room, on your body by putting it in your pocket or bra or holding it in your hand while meditating. If you don't want to buy extra crystals, you can work with the ones you already have, especially clear quartz, by telling the crystal what you want it to do.

We don't recommend placing blue lace agate or obsidian in the bath, but you can place them in your bathroom or around your tub to achieve a similar effect.

Essential Oils

Previously, we discussed using frankincense and lavender to support your root chakra. You can continue working with these oils or try cypress oil. Cypress oil comes from the cypress tree, an evergreen perennial, and is great for boosting your energy. It can be applied topically or diffused to lift your spirits. Try adding a drop or two to your favorite unscented lotion before applying. When diffused, cypress oil can be very grounding and invigorating, helping to center and energize you.

To support your throat chakra, try working with sage essential oil. Sage is known as a master herb, and this is where sage essential oil comes from. It was considered to be sacred in ancient Greek and Roman times and, like cypress, is also an evergreen shrub. Sage can help you feel more mindful and positive. Together these two oils act as a powerhouse in helping you find the courage to ask for help and seek out the most supportive people in your life.

Sage can be applied topically or diffused, but because it is a common herb to cook with, you can also enjoy its benefits by incorporating it into your meals. Sage goes well with many meat, pasta, and veggie dishes.

Another fun thing to do with sage is called smudging. Smudging involves cleansing a space or person of unwanted energy. You can purchase smudging sticks or bundles from your local metaphysical shop or make your own with dried sage. Light the sage, then blow out the flame so the herb is smoking. Then use your hand to waft the smoke over the area you want to cleanse of negative energy.

Like clear quartz is considered a master crystal, lavender is considered a master essential oil. If you don't want to purchase essential oils to correspond to each chakra, we recommend starting with lavender because it works to cleanse and balance all the chakras. Remember to set an intention as to what you want to achieve by using the oil, whether you are diffusing it or applying it topically.

There are also many ways to use the lavender plant including making a tea from the dried flowers, planting some in your garden or a planter, and using it in salads or to decorate cakes or cookies.

Journal Prompt

In your releasing journal, write any fears you might have about finding support on your journey to be the happiest version of you. Ask yourself:

- · What fears do I have around finding support?
- · What is preventing me from finding support?

In your gratitude journal, or on the page provided, write as if you have found the support you visualized in your meditation. Write about how thankful you are to have that support. If you need help getting started, ask yourself, "How do I want to feel when I have the support I need?"

Summary

Remember, you're not in this life alone. Having supportive people you can count on is an important step in your journey, as is letting go of the relationships that are no longer fulfilling for you. Whichever tools you feel are helping you the most, whether it's crystals, essential oils, yoga poses, meditations, or affirmations, take full advantage of them as you continue to work through the chapters in this book.

Don't be afraid to step out of your comfort zone. Up until this chapter, you've been mostly working on your own, so this is a big step. Take a deep breath and remember the quote from Michelle Obama that we shared in Chapter 3: "Just try new things. Don't be afraid. Step out of your comfort zones and soar, all right?"

You've got this!

Action Step

It can be difficult to ask for help, but it's so worth it. Start by saying, "Hi." This week, as you work with your tools and gain confidence in your ability to find support, think about where you will look to make connections with like-minded people. Is it an online social community, like a Facebook group, an in-person community meet-up, or something fun like a new hobby group?

If connecting with people online isn't your thing, call a friend or make an appointment to see your doctor so you can learn about the groups available in your local area.

5

Experimenting with New Tools

"Learn something new. Try something different. Convince yourself that you have no limits."

—*Brian Tracy*

You have no limits!

Let that sink in for a moment . . .

If you have no limits that means you can do anything you want, including living the life of your dreams. What an amazing thought. The possibilities are endless. We hope, at this point of the book, you are starting to feel less stuck and more open to the possibilities that are available to you.

We've already given you many options when it comes to tools you can use as you work on becoming a happier version of yourself. As you meet people that are aligned with and supportive of this new version of yourself, you will learn about the tools they like to use. You'll be exposed to even more tools you can try. The possibilities are endless!

You may also find that once you are comfortable with the tools in this book, you'll become curious about what else is out there. Or maybe some of the tools you started with won't resonate with you anymore and you'll want to try something different. That's a natural part of the process, and in this chapter, we'll be covering the usual tools as well as some new bonus tools for you to try, if you're so inclined.

The great thing about the tools we've shared so far, as well as the new tools we'll be sharing, is they all act as a way for you to gain a further understanding of yourself and what you truly want in your life. If you don't like a tool we recommend, there are plenty more to choose from.

Chakras

The chakras that come into play during this stage of your transformation are the sacral chakra and the solar plexus chakra. To be open to experimenting with new tools, you'll need to keep an open mind. This requires creativity and self-mastery. It's time to step more fully into your personal power.

Remember that the sacral chakra is associated with creativity. Creativity is important when working with new tools. Not only will you come up with new ways to use the tools you already love, but you'll also need to keep an open mind when learning about new tools you can experiment with.

The sacral chakra also helps us connect with our emotions. This is important, because your goal when experimenting with new tools (or new ways to use old tools) is to bring more happiness into your life. A blockage in the sacral chakra can cause our emotions to run out of control resulting in overreactions.

We'll share some additional tools with you in this chapter to help balance your sacral chakra before you start experimenting with new tools, but if your experiments don't feel happy to you, simply move on to the next tool or continue using the tools that already bring you joy.

When our solar plexus chakra isn't balanced, we can become very controlling, making it difficult for us to be open to new experiences. This isn't good when it comes to experimenting with new tools. The exercises in this chapter will help you open up to the idea of experimenting with new tools as well as encourage confidence in your ability to know when a tool is right for you.

Yoga Pose

Abdominal Lift
The abdominal lift is a great pose for improving the health of the solar plexus, because it stimulates the solar plexus and tones the abdomen. This exercise targets the physical location of your solar plexus chakra.

Step 1: Stand with your feet a bit wider than hip-width apart. Bend forward slightly, resting your hands on your thighs with your knees slightly bent.

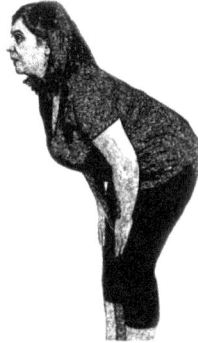

Step 2: With your head parallel to the ground and your face turned towards the ground, breathe in deeply then exhale thoroughly. Pull your abdomen in and up towards the back of your spine so that it forms a hollow. Hold this for as long as possible.

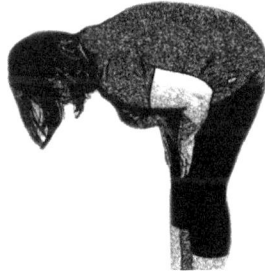

Step 3: Repeat the inhale and exhale as many times as you like. When you're ready to come out of the pose, return to an upright position, inhaling and exhaling long and slow.

Affirmations

The affirmations in this chapter focus on boosting your confidence so you'll be comfortable trying new things. Try saying the affirmations while looking at yourself in the mirror.

· I allow myself to try something different.
· I flow into happiness.
· I accept expansion every day.

Meditation

This meditation is all about using your new support network to help you discover more tools you can use to continue your journey towards a happier life. Sit or lie in a comfortable position with your eyes closed. Focus on your breath while you take deep breaths in through your nose and out through your mouth.

Picture a wonderful support group around you. This can be people you already know, or people you are hoping will come into your life when you need them most. They are here for you now, ready to help and support you.

Turn to one of the people you are visualizing and ask them what new tool they recommend for you. You may not see or hear anything while you are meditating, but be on the lookout for messages as you go about your day and week. Sometimes messages arrive when we least expect them.

Now ask if there is a tool you already use that you can use in a different way. Continue to meditate, observing what's happening in your mind's eye and what messages you are receiving. When you are ready, open your eyes and take a deep breath to bring yourself back to the here and now. Remember to make notes about what you experienced.

If you don't feel like meditating today, try some doodles, or get out your pencil crayons and color. Remember, there are extra coloring pages at the back of the book. If you're using markers, you might want to place a piece of cardboard under the coloring page, so the marker doesn't bleed through.

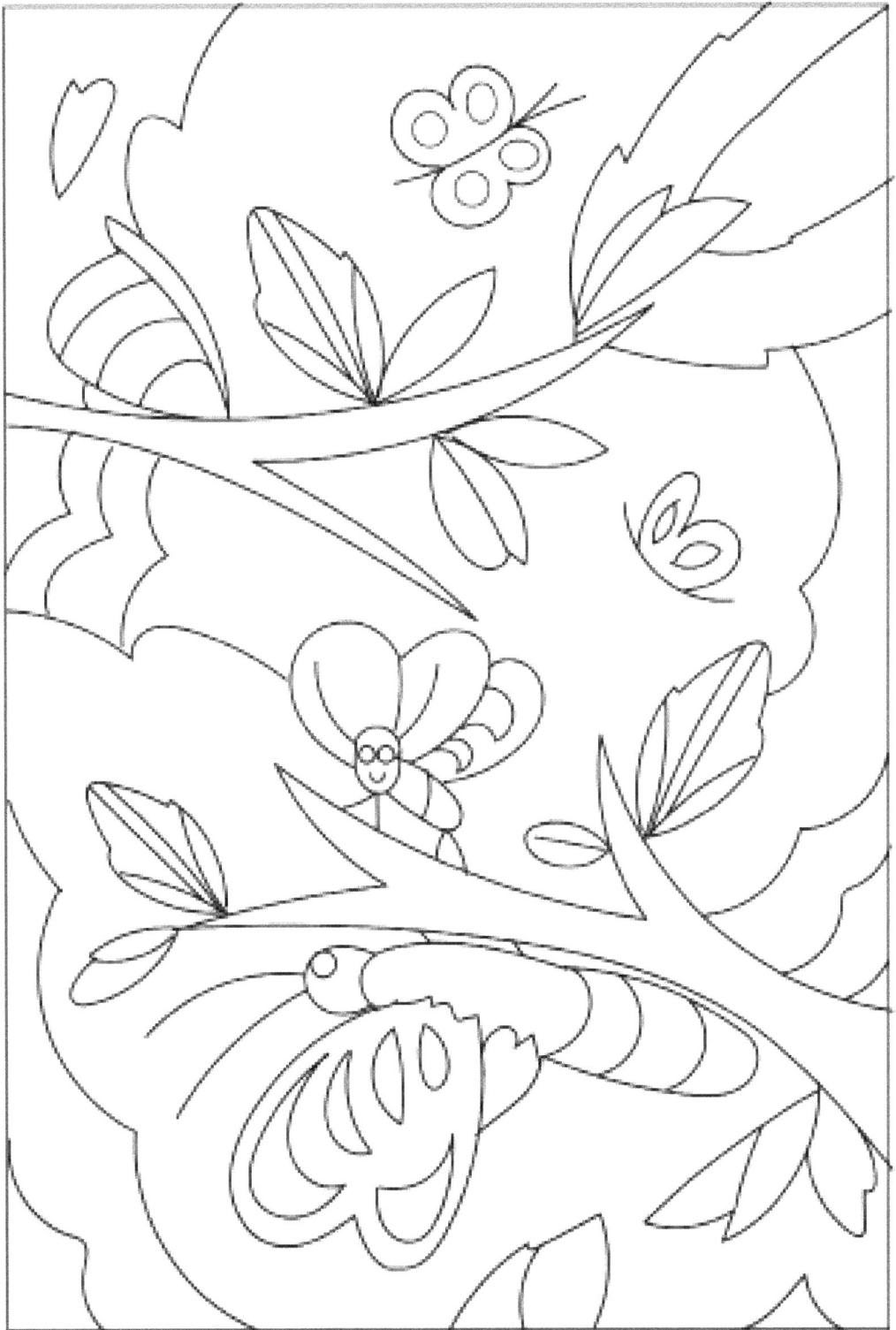

Use this page to **DOODLE**. If using markers, you may want to place extra paper or a piece of cardboard under this page to prevent bleed through. Have fun!

Crystals

We've already mentioned three crystals that are great for the solar plexus chakra: citrine, amber, and tiger eye. You can continue working with any of these. If you'd like to try something new, aventurine can also be helpful. Green aventurine is a type of quartz that contains mica and other minerals that give it a beautiful green color. It can be found in Africa, the US, and India.

Commonly known as a stone of personal growth, green aventurine has a soothing energy and can be used to help with many emotional issues, but we chose it here because of its ability to help with new growth—perfect for supporting you as you experiment with new tools. You can wear aventurine, place it near you in your home, carry it with you in your purse, and, because it is a type of quartz, you can bathe with it.

For supporting your sacral chakra, once again, you can use carnelian as recommended in Chapter 3, but if you want to try another crystal, moonstone is also excellent. Moonstone is named for its moon-like sheen and has an opalescent quality. It comes mostly from Sri Lanka and India, but it can also be found in the US, Brazil, and Australia.

Moonstone is a wonderful crystal to help with sacral chakra support because it promotes creative energy and healing: two important attributes when it comes to experimenting with new tools. Because of its association with the moon, it also has a very feminine and loving energy. Both aventurine and moonstone can be found in jewellery, but you are encouraged to use them in whichever way you enjoy the most, whether that is wearing them, placing them in a spot where you will see them every day, or meditating with them.

Essential Oils

Ylang ylang is a great oil for supporting both the sacral chakra and the solar plexus chakra, so you can continue using that one if you decided to try it in Chapter 3. And because lavender is great for supporting all the chakras, you can also use lavender.

If you're interested in trying some new oils to help you as you experiment with new tools, we recommend jasmine for the sacral chakra and lemon for the solar plexus chakra. Jasmine essential oil comes from the flowers of the jasmine plant usually found in tropical climates.

The health benefits of jasmine include easing depression, preventing infection, and even acting as an aphrodisiac. Because it is known as an arousing oil, it is very effective at relieving the symptoms associated with depression. This arousing effect will also stimulate your creativity when it comes to experimenting with your tools.

As you may have guessed, lemon essential oil comes from lemons and is also a stimulating oil. Its fresh lemon scent is energizing and refreshing. It has been used in everything from skin care to laundry and furniture polish. While lemon is known to be a mood booster, it's lesser known that it's also an immune booster.

As recommended in previous chapters, you can use your oils by diffusing them or diluting them in a carrier oil such as coconut oil and applying topically. Because this chapter is all about experimenting with new tools or using existing tools in new ways, try a method of working with essential oils you haven't tried before.

For the lemon oil, buy a fresh lemon and use its juice and/or peel in some baking or to flavor your tea or water. For a twist on traditional diffusing, give yourself a mini facial by placing a couple of drops of essential oil in a bowl of hot water and draping a towel over your head, like a tent, to catch the steam.

As long as you are being safe with your oils and using them as directed, you can be creative with how you use them and in what combinations. We discuss combining essential oils more in Chapter 7.

Journal Prompt

When writing in your releasing journal, we want you to ask yourself what fears you have around trying new tools. Keep writing about these fears until you feel them lessening. It's okay if you don't know why you have these fears. Ask the universe to take them away.

Once you've written about all the fears you have around experimenting with new tools, you can rip up your paper and throw it away or safely burn it.

In your gratitude journal, we'd like you to write about all the tools you are thankful for. There are so many different things to try and many different ways to use them that we know you'll find something you love.

Write about how you are grateful for the opportunity to learn more about these simple tools that can help improve the health of your chakras and your overall well-being.

Summary

Like a butterfly coming out of its cocoon for the first time, you are learning to spread your wings and fly. Part of the process of transforming your life to be happier and more true to yourself is trying new things that will support you on your journey.

If you're not sure what to try, that's okay. Ask your support network what tools they enjoy using and what things make them happy every day. We've suggested some of our favorite tools in the action step, but you can also find many more by researching online.

Action Step

Choose one new tool and get familiar with it. If you're not sure what to try, here are some suggestions from some of our favorite things.

Oracle Cards
Oracle cards can be used to receive messages from the universe or other higher power you believe in. Oracle card decks come in various sizes with forty-four cards being common. Most people choose their deck based on the artwork. They are fun and easy to use and usually come with a guidebook that goes deeper into the message of each card.

Color Therapy
There are many forms of color therapy. For the purposes of this book, we refer to color therapy as using the colors that represent the chakras in your everyday life. For example, in this chapter we discussed the sacral and solar plexus chakras, so if you want to work with colors to improve the health of those chakras, you can wear lots of orange and yellow, color with orange and yellow, eat orange and yellow foods, and visualize oranges and yellows around you as you meditate.

Finger Labyrinth
A finger labyrinth is a small version of a walking labyrinth or maze. Instead of walking the maze, with a finger labyrinth, you trace the path to the center of the labyrinth with your finger. The labyrinth is usually carved in wood and can be used for relaxation, meditation, or prayer.

Candles
Lighting a candle is a quick and easy way to provide a relaxing ambience. You can also meditate with candles: simply light a candle then sit in a comfortable position and watch the

flame. You will see the flame waver and flicker, and you might even see some shapes appear. This is a great meditation technique if you have trouble calming your mind, because it gives you something to focus on.

Pendulums
Pendulums are a lot fun. They are usually made from a crystal that is pointed at one end and suspended from a chain at the other end, but they can be any kind of weighted object. Even a favorite necklace will work. Pendulums can be used to answer yes or no questions and help you further understand your intuition.

6

Finding What Works for You

"Life is so much simpler when you stop explaining yourself to people and just do what works for you."

—healthyplace.com

Part of becoming your happiest self is forgetting about what everyone else tells you to do. That's a recipe for getting stuck. We do what other people think we should do and we get so used to doing what everyone else wants that soon we have no idea what we want anymore. The only way you can transform your life is to understand what you want.

Once you understand what you really want and what makes you truly happy, it's easier to make choices that reflect that. The same goes for discovering the tools you want to use on your journey. Just because we (the authors) have certain things that we enjoy using and have worked well for us, doesn't mean those same things are going to work well for you.

Think back to our butterfly analogy. When butterflies are learning to fly, they use their instincts to discover how to flap their wings in order to get to their intended destination. Feeling comfortable with yourself and your choices is like learning to fly. Follow your gut instincts. Even if it's been a long time since you've understood what makes you happy, there's still a good chance you remember what that feels like. Feel into those happy feelings and follow your intuition when making choices based on how you want to live your life.

If thinking about what makes you happy feels frustrating and overwhelming, we want you to know this is perfectly normal. When you've spent your life doing what other people want you to do, it takes time and practice to listen to yourself again to know what you want and what makes you happy.

Be gentle with yourself and relax. You have lots of time to try all the tools and exercises we've described and make them your own so you can use them in the way that works best for you. If you're feeling overwhelmed then go back to working with one tool each week. There's no pressure to do things a certain way. This is all about you and learning to live your happiest life, so there's no right way, just your way!

Chakras

When listening to your intuition and learning to do things your way, you will rely on your third eye and heart chakras. Remember from the introduction, that the third eye chakra is located on your forehead, between your eyebrows. The third eye chakra helps us see things clearly, trust our intuition, and become more self aware. A blocked third eye chakra, on the other hand, can lead to paranoia, closed mindedness, mental illness, anxiety, and depression.

A big part of knowing what you want is trusting your intuition, which is why, for this part of your transformation, it's important to have a clear and balanced third eye chakra. When you're relaxed and at peace with yourself, it's easier to listen to you intuition. This is where your heart chakra comes in—to be happy with yourself, you must also love yourself.

A blocked or unbalanced heart chakra can cause you to stuff your emotions, and when you stuff your emotions, you prevent yourself from feeling the good feelings too. Emotions are a natural part of being human and they are a necessary way we receive feedback from ourselves and others. When you're free to experience all your emotions, you can truly love and appreciate yourself and others.

When your heart chakra is clear, you will feel deeply connected to yourself and the energy around you. This connection will help you feel confident in doing what's right for you as you work through this transformation to a happier version of yourself. In addition to experiencing great self-love, an open heart chakra can help you feel more compassionate towards others, have an easier time with relationships, and be more forgiving and accepting.

Yoga Pose

Eye Exercises

As you may have guessed, eye exercises help improve the health of the third eye chakra. Not only do these exercises stimulate the third eye chakra, but they also improve eye circulation and strengthen the muscles around the eyes.

Step 1: Stand or sit in a comfortable position. Warm your hands by rubbing them together, then gently put them over your eyes.

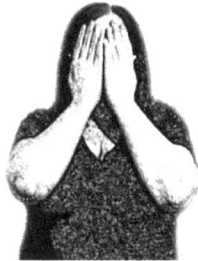

Step 2: Gradually open your fingers to let light in. Then open your eyes and lower your hands.

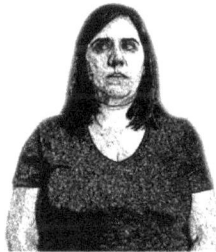

Step 3: Visualize a clock in front of you. Look at the twelve o'clock position then down to six o'clock five times. Close your eyes and squeeze them tight. Open your eyes when you're ready.

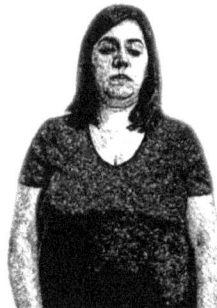

Step 4: Now do the same thing, but look at the three o'clock position and the nine o'clock position five times. Once again, close your eyes and squeeze them tight.

Step 5: Repeat Step 4, but now look from one o'clock to seven o'clock five times. Then squeeze your eyes tight, and open them when you are ready.

Step 6: Gently place your hands over your eyes as you did in Step 1. Remove your hands when you are ready.

Affirmations

Try these affirmations to help you trust your intuition and do what works best for you:

- I trust my intuition.
- I'm happy being me.
- I notice what makes me feel good.

Through the course of this book, we have suggested various ways you can use these affirmations. For this chapter, use your affirmations in your favorite ways. Here's a reminder of some of the things we've suggested:

- Write affirmations on sticky notes and post them on your computer screen or bathroom mirror.
- Use your journal to write your favorite affirmations over and over on the page.
- Record yourself saying your favorite affirmation.
- Create some art including one or more affirmations.

Meditation

Often, when we do things that don't make us happy, it's because we feel like we "should" do these things based on what we see other people doing or what other people have told us. For this meditation, we are going to practice letting go of the "shoulds".

Sit or lie in a comfortable position. Close your eyes and take three deep breaths. Imagine all the times you felt you "should" do something. Visualize those things floating away. You can even imagine the word "should" floating away if that is easier. Let go of all those shoulds and expectations that come from other people.

Now, visualize the things you want. See yourself doing all the things that are important to you. Feel how happy you are. Sit with this happiness for a while, letting it fill you with joy. When you're ready, take three deep breaths, and open your eyes.

You may want to grab your journal and make some notes about how happy you felt and what you were doing or what tools you were using that made you feel that way. You can refer back to your notes when you're having a bad day. Do this meditation any time you are feeling anxious about feeling like you "should" do something. Just let it go!

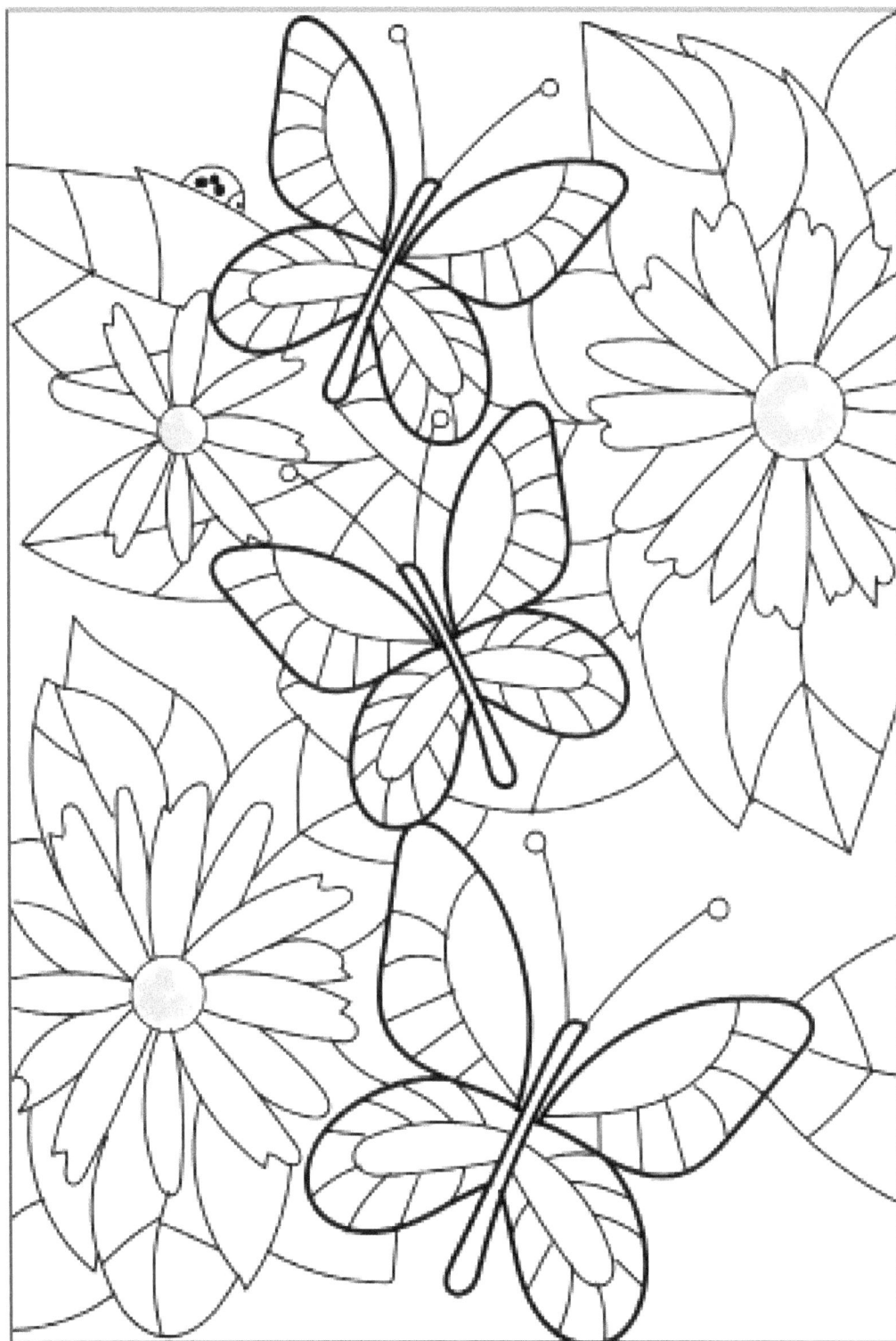

Use this page to **DOODLE**. If using markers, you may want to place extra paper or a piece of cardboard under this page to prevent bleed through. Have fun!

Crystals

One of the best crystals for working with the third eye chakra is amethyst. Amethyst is a purple stone from the quartz family. It's considered a semi-precious stone and can be found in many locations around the world. Because it's from the quartz family, it's also safe to use in bath water if that is your preferred way to work with crystals.

Throughout history, amethyst has been known for its powers to stimulate and soothe the mind. Because of these properties, amethyst is an excellent stone for helping you become more connected to yourself and your intuition. A fun thing to try when working with amethyst to open your third eye chakra, is to lie down and place the amethyst on your third eye chakra. Relax and practice deep breathing while visualizing your third eye chakra opening. Visualizing it as another eye can help.

For the heart chakra, one of the best crystals is rose quartz. As the name suggests, rose quartz is also from the quartz family. It's a beautiful light pink. Rose quartz has been called "the heart stone" and "the universal stone of love" because it encourages love and compassion for the self and others. Rose quartz is also an aphrodisiac, calming and reassuring, and helps promote a good night's sleep.

The focus of this chapter is finding what works for you. If you already have some favorite methods of working with your crystals, continue using them. If, on the other hand, you're still looking for a method that works for you or you just haven't connected to your crystals yet, that's totally okay. Choose one of the methods we've suggested previously or focus on what works for you!

Essential Oils

Patchouli is a great oil for working with the third eye chakra. It has a warm, musky scent that is commonly associated with the hippie generation. The patchouli plant belongs to the same family as the aromatic plants that produce lavender and sage. A fun fact about patchouli is that it was used to scent fabrics in the 1800s to prevent insects from ruining them.

In addition to being anti-inflammatory and antidepressant, patchouli is also grounding and balancing, two much needed qualities when working on your third eye chakra. When the third eye first starts to open and you begin listening to your intuition more, it can be easy to feel overwhelmed and unsure of what you are experiencing. Physical symptoms like dizziness and light-headedness are common when this happens. Staying grounded and balanced will minimize these symptoms and help you trust your experiences.

For supporting the heart chakra, we recommend clary sage essential oil. Clary sage is a flowering herb found in the Mediteranean and has a lovely fresh and flowery scent. It's great for stress reduction and, like patchouli, it's a natural antidepressant. Clary sage can also be used for menstrual and menopausal support. Dilute the oil with a carrier oil, such as coconut oil, and apply topically over your heart.

Since this chapter is all about finding the tools and routines that work for you, choose your favorite way of working with essential oils. Remember to dilute your oils if applying them topically and check the bottle for other safety precautions.

As we mentioned before, you certainly don't need to buy all these oils. Lavender is a great support for all the chakras. These are just options.

Journal Prompt

When thinking about finding what works for you and a way to be happy in your life, we want you to think about what hasn't worked in the past. It's time to let go of that way of doing things. In your releasing journal, answer the question:

· What hasn't worked for me in the past?

When you're done pouring out your heart and soul about all the things that haven't worked to make you happy, remember to let those thoughts go. You can tear up the paper, safely burn it, or just leave it in your journal and visualize all those things being released as you turn the page. Ask the universe or other higher power you believe in to help you let them go.

For your gratitude journal prompt, we want you to flip things around and write about what has worked for you, either in the past or right now. In your gratitude journal, answer the question:

· What am I grateful for that's helping me live a happier life?

Summary

You are starting to own your happiness and feel what it takes to live your happiest life. Like a butterfly learning to fly for the first time, you are following your intuition and doing what makes sense to you.

Practice appreciating yourself and the things that make you happy. Over time, you'll find you no longer have to think about what makes you happy, but you'll instinctively know. Take time throughout your day to sit quietly with yourself and listen to your intuition.

Action Step

Pick your favorite tool or practice, something that makes you insanely happy, and do it every day this week. Put it on your calendar or set a reminder so you don't forget. You are worth it and you deserve to do things that make you happy!

7

Making Time for Yourself

"Making time for yourself is an art, and like every art, it requires practice."
—*Christina Katz*

A common theme among women is that they feel guilty for taking time for themselves. Not only is taking time for yourself an important step in living your happiest life, but it's also necessary for your survival. We all need time to ourselves to reflect, relax, and recharge. If you're not doing this every day, even for five minutes, you are going to have a harder time finding your happiness.

One of the reasons it's so challenging for women to make time for themselves is that, as caregivers, they often put others first. This includes children, other family members, friends, coworkers, and neighbors. It's easy to get in the habit of putting everyone else first, but this does you no good. The happier you are, the better your relationships will be. Look at the classic example from the airlines: In an emergency situation, you're no good to anyone if you don't put on your own oxygen mask first. Think of taking care of yourself as putting on your oxygen mask.

A big help when making time for yourself is creating a habit or routine of caring for yourself. Let the people close to you know that at a certain time every day, you will be taking ten minutes (or whatever length of time you choose) for yourself. Then make sure you do that so they will understand you are serious. Letting people know ahead of time can help ease the guilt you feel for taking that time, and it can also help hold you accountable for following through and actually taking a few minutes for yourself every day.

At this point in your transformation journey, you should be feeling excited for all the progress you've made so far. You're learning what makes you happy and setting healthy boundaries in your relationships, and you've been introduced to many tools that can help you along the way. Now it's up to you to make a commitment to yourself and continue taking the necessary time to feed your soul.

Chakras

When it comes to making time for yourself and maintaining your connection to your body, mind, and soul so you can continue to live your best life, you're going to need the whole chakra system working at its best. But first, there is one chakra we haven't discussed yet, and that's because it was important to get your other chakras balanced and cleared first. Now that you've been working on those chakras, let's talk about the crown chakra.

The crown chakra helps you connect with a higher power. A balanced crown chakra helps keep the other chakras balanced too. When the crown chakra is functioning at its best, you are able to achieve enlightenment and extreme clarity. Think of the crown chakra as the point in between your mind, body, and soul that also connects you to the energy of the universe around you.

When your crown chakra isn't balanced, you may feel like you are walking around in a fog. You will also feel uninspired and disconnected from the world around you. While it's not necessary to have all the chakras clear and balanced before working on your crown chakra, it often happens that way because of the crown chakra's connection to universal energy. As you learn more about your own energy and what each chakra's job is, you will know when certain chakras require you to spend more time balancing and clearing them.

The chakras work best in connection with each other. It's important to maintain the health of all your chakras to keep your body, mind, and spirit at their best. Each chakra is responsible for certain parts of the physical body as well as the mind and spirit, so physical symptoms will often be your first clue that something isn't quite right in one or more of your chakras.

Keeping your crown chakra, and all the rest of your chakras, balanced will help you make time for yourself, because you will start to see noticeable differences in how you feel when your chakras are balanced and clear. The only way to keep the chakras clear and balanced is to spend a little time working with them each day. The more you do things for yourself and the health of your chakras, the better you'll feel and the more you'll want to keep your chakras balanced.

It's natural positive reinforcement!

Yoga Pose

Visualize

Many people don't realize that visualization is a key component of yoga and has been around as long as the ancient practice. The meditations we've shared in this book are visualizations— pictures in your mind.

A fun visualization for the crown chakra is to imagine it's a lotus flower sitting at the crown of your head. Decide before you start the visualization how many petals your flower has. It can be any number you choose, more petals if you have more time. Or you can choose seven petals, one for each chakra.

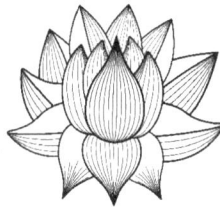

Start with the lotus blossom closed. Take three deep breaths. Now, each time you take a breath, imagine the flower opening a petal. Continue until all the petals are open. Relax with the flower open for as long as you like. Before you're done visualizing, you'll want to close the petals slightly because having a wide open crown chakra can lead to its overactivity which will leave you feeling run down and vulnerable to physical and mental ailments.

When you're ready, reverse the visualization. With each breath, picture a petal on the lotus blossom closing part way. You don't want to close it all the way, because a closed crown chakra will cut you off from connecting with universal and spiritual energy. Continue visualizing each petal partially closing until the entire lotus blossom is partially closed.

When you're ready, take three deep breaths, and open your eyes.

Affirmations

Affirmations take very little time and can be said to yourself throughout the day. They are a quick and easy way to make time for yourself. Say one every time you're looking at yourself in the bathroom mirror while washing your hands. Here are some to try:

- · I am stable, safe, and secure.
- · I make time to care for myself.
- · I am establishing a healthy routine.

If you have more than just a couple of minutes, using your affirmations in different ways can help you remember them. For example, if you are someone who learns best by reading, you'll want to write several affirmations on sticky notes or recipe cards so you can read them throughout the day. You can also refer to the affirmations list at the end of the book and choose random affirmations. We guarantee you will intuitively find the affirmations you need for the day.

Meditation

There are many ways to meditate besides visualizing and deep breathing. Here are some simple meditations you can do in just five minutes or less:

Cloud Gazing
Go outside, look up, and see what you notice about the clouds in the sky. Are they drifting, or stationary? If you have time, find a comfortable spot on the grass and see what unique shapes you can find in the clouds. This is a really fun thing to do with the kids in your life too!

Leaf Dancing
This is another simple way to meditate. Go to a local park or walk around your neighborhood and find some trees with leaves that are gently moving to and fro. Take a few minutes to quietly observe how the leaves wave in the breeze. Take as little or as much time as you want.

Candle Burning
Staring at a candle is another easy way to meditate that doesn't take long. Light your favorite candle and stare at the flame. As the flame flickers you may get a message from your higher power or see a shape in the flame.

Walking
Walking is also a form of meditation, especially when you're able to go by yourself. The trick is to focus your mind rather than let it wander. A wandering mind is great when you are trying to work out problems and get new ideas, but when you're meditating, you want to clear your mind. If you find random thoughts popping into your head, just let them go.

To meditate while walking, focus on your steps. If you can walk barefoot in your backyard, this is the ultimate walking meditation, because you will strengthen your connection to the earth by feeling the ground beneath your feet. If this isn't possible, you can still focus on the earth with each step you take, allowing you to relax and clear your mind.

Remember, coloring and doodling are also great ways to meditate. If you plan to use markers on your coloring page, remember to insert a piece of cardboard under the page you are working on to prevent bleed-through to pages underneath.

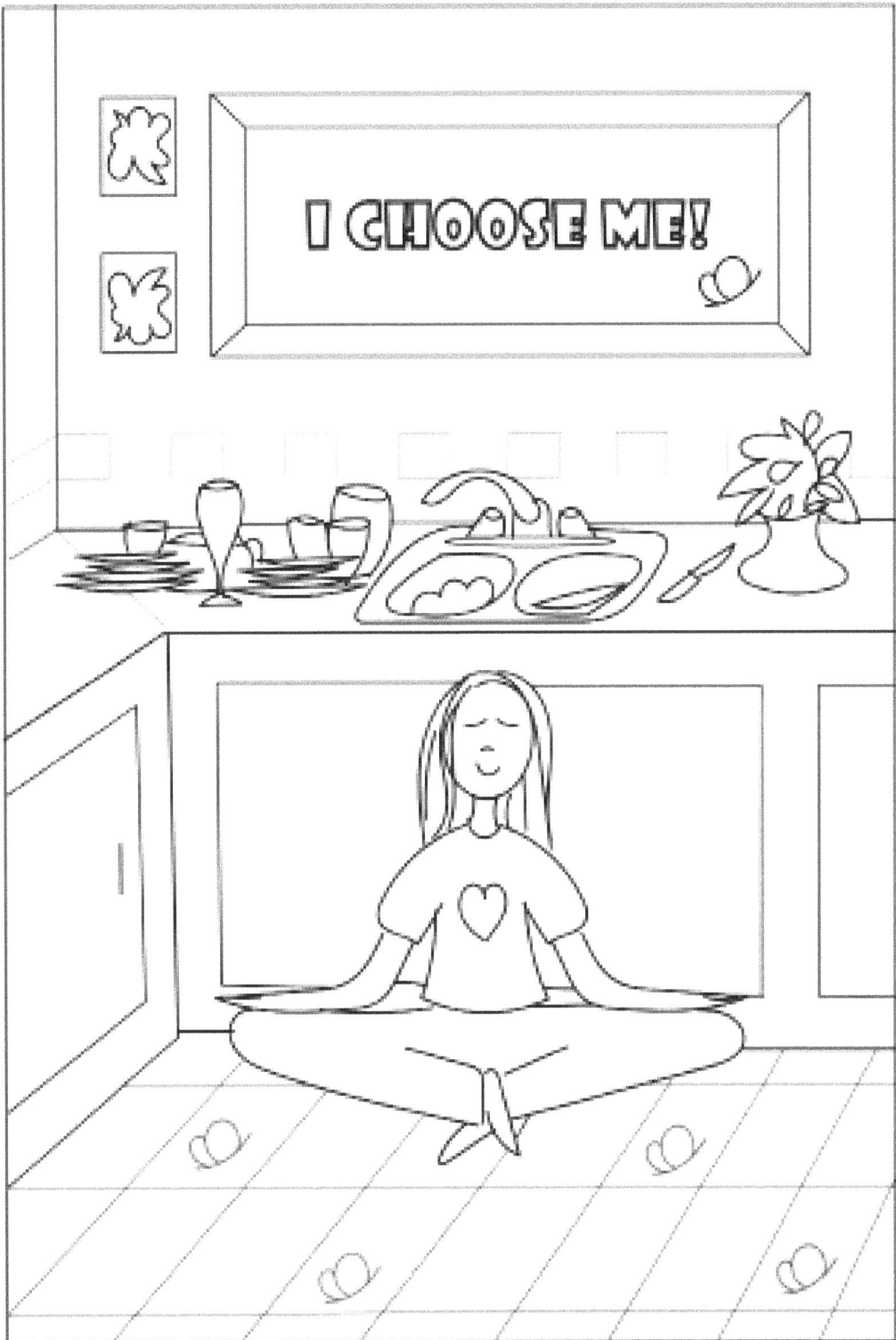

Use this page to **DOODLE**. If using markers, you may want to place extra paper or a piece of cardboard under this page to prevent bleed through. Have fun!

Crystals

We've mentioned before that clear quartz is one of the most powerful crystals. You can use it for almost anything you can imagine. That's why we think it's the perfect crystal for working with the crown chakra. You may want to hold it in your hand while doing the lotus blossom visualization.

As a quick review, clear quartz represents clarity and, for that reason, is excellent for clearing the mind and enhancing spiritual receptiveness. It's a healing and protective stone that is inexpensive and easy to find in stores.

Clear quartz can be used to quickly clear and balance the crown chakra. It's also wonderful for clearing the lower chakras. Use it while meditating, use it as a wand, focusing the areas of the body where the chakras are, or wear it as jewelry to protect and clear your chakras throughout the day.

Another crystal that can be used to work with the entire chakra system is super seven. This stone is sometimes called the sacred seven and, as the name suggests, contains seven different crystals:

· Amethyst,
· Cacoxenite,
· Clear quartz,
· Goethite,
· Rutite,
· Smokey quartz, and
· Lepidocrocite.

Each mineral in the super seven stone is said to represent each of the seven chakras, so this makes it a wonderful stone to use when you want to work with the entire chakra system. It can be a difficult stone to find.

Super seven is an excellent crystal to meditate with because it eases passage to the unconscious mind. It also helps you understand your life purpose and what is holding you back. Seeing and removing boundaries to live your life purpose is a major part of living your life on purpose and becoming the happiest version of yourself.

Essential Oils

Lavender is an excellent oil for promoting peace and calmness, essential qualities when working on balancing your crown chakra. As we've mentioned before, lavender is a universal oil, which means it can be used to balance and clear all the chakras.

An easy way to use lavender for the crown chakra is to diffuse it while you sleep or dilute it and rub some on your crown before going to bed. This will help you connect with the energy of the universe and your higher power while you sleep.

A fun thing to do if you have more than one essential oil in your collection of spiritual tools, is creating your own essential oil blend. You can do this by combining different oils in your diffuser, or mixing different oils in a base of coconut oil or another carrier oil. You can create a chakra blend that combines a drop of oil for each chakra.

If you're not sure if your oils will smell nice together, you can test this using a cotton ball or Kleenex first. Add a drop of each oil to the cotton ball and after you add each oil, leave it for a few minutes, then go back to it and see how it smells. Make notes as you go, so you'll know which oils smell nice together.

Citrus oils typically blend well with florals, woody, minty, and spicy oils, while earthy oils tend to go well with musky, minty and spicy oils. It might take a bit of experimenting to see which combinations you like the best, which is why we recommend using a cotton ball at first. When you know what combinations you like, then you can diffuse them or make a roller bottle with a carrier oil.

Journal Prompt

Why does it always seem so hard to make time for ourselves? This is the question we'd like you to ponder in your releasing journal.

Write this question at the top of a page in your releasing journal:

· What is stopping me from making time for myself?

Then write all the excuses you use for not making time for yourself. When you're done remember to let go of all your negative thoughts. You can do this by ripping up the page you wrote on, burning it or even burying it in the ground—whatever feels right to you.

In your gratitude journal, we'd like to you to list all the things you are grateful for when you make time for yourself. At the top of a page in your gratitude journal write:

· When I make time for myself I feel . . .

Now, write down all the reasons you are grateful for time to yourself. If you don't get much time for yourself right now, you can write as if you are at a point in the future where you do get the time to yourself that you need. What are you grateful for?

Summary

Like a butterfly venturing out more and more on their own, you are learning to take some much needed time for yourself. Even a few minutes to yourself each day will help you feel relaxed and rejuvenated and better able to face the day from a happier place.

Not only do you deserve time to yourself, but it's also a necessary step in living your happiest life. The only way we can know what truly makes us happy is to spend time with ourselves reflecting.

Action Step

Practice putting yourself first by scheduling time for yourself on your calendar each day this month. Go ahead, grab your calendar—we'll wait!

8

Maintaining Your Freedom

"It's not selfish to love yourself, take care of yourself, and to make your happiness a priority. It's necessary."

—*Mandy Hale*

Congratulations, you've done it! You've freed your inner butterfly! But the thing with negative behaviors and patterns is, they took most of your life to create. Don't be surprised if you find them sneaking back into your life from time to time. That's perfectly normal and that's why it's important to practice the new skills you've learned.

We hope, at this point in the book, you've removed some of the limits you put on yourself in the past and are learning to set healthy boundaries in your life. Even if you have many people that depend on you, you still need to find time to do things for yourself. This is how you "maintain your freedom" and continue to live your happiest life.

While we may not have the luxury of flying wherever we want whenever we want, like butterflies, we do have the ability to set limits on other people's demands on us. You can and should say "no" when you feel you need to. You also have the ability to choose activities that bring you joy. To enjoy your new found happiness, you need to keep up the good habit of taking time for yourself. Choose to do things that make you happy and enjoy them every day.

Chakras

Throughout this book, we've given you an introduction to the main chakras in the chakra system and provided some simple exercises you can do to balance and clear them. The more you work with your chakras, the more you will know which chakras need your attention. You will likely start to feel this intuitively as well as experience the physical and mental symptoms that present themselves when your chakras aren't balanced.

Refer to the references and recommended resources section for books that provide more information about the chakras as well as some of the other things we've discussed herein. An easy way to keep your chakras balanced and clear is to work on the whole system at once. This is also a great place to start when you're not sure which specific chakra needs work.

When your chakra system is balanced, you will feel healthy and energetic. You'll also notice your relationships with other people are healthy, and you can easily express yourself. Your intuition will become stronger and you'll have an easier time relying on it as you begin to feel more connected to a higher power and live more in line with your greater purpose. When this happens you'll experience a lot more happiness in your life too!

Yoga Pose

Savasana (Corpse Pose)

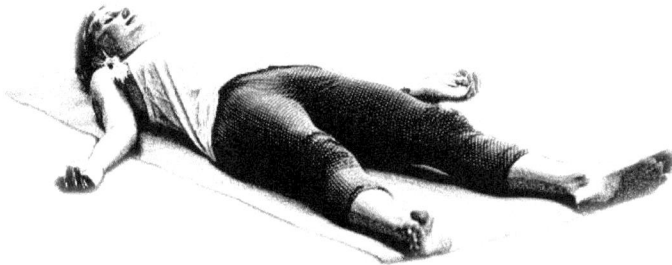

Savasana, commonly called corpse pose, is simply lying down. You can do this on a yoga mat or a comfortable spot on the floor. Let your arms and legs relax and fall to the side. Feel your body getting heavy and sinking into the floor.

Close your eyes and focus on your breath while in this position. Try to breathe deeply into your belly and remember to exhale fully. Any time you feel your thoughts wander, focus on your breath. You can also focus on each chakra to help keep your mind from wandering.

Start with your root chakra at the base of your pelvis. Visualize its color, red, and see it spinning freely in a clockwise motion. Then move to the sacral chakra. See the beautiful orange that represents the sacral chakra, and again, see it spinning freely. Take as much time as you need to visualize each chakra.

From the sacral chakra, move to your solar plexus chakra. Here you will see a bright yellow light while your chakra is spinning freely. At the heart chakra, visualize a light green energy. Some people also see pink at the heart chakra. Feel into whatever you see. Next is the throat chakra. See the chakra spinning freely and a light blue energy radiating from it.

At the third eye chakra visualize an indigo light and your third eye chakra spinning freely. When you're ready, move to the crown chakra. The crown chakra is usually associated with a violet light, but many people also see a white light here, representing your connection to the divine. Once you've visualized each chakra, imagine a healing light surrounding you. This can be any color. Stay in this position as long as you like.

When you're ready, focus on your breath. Take three deep breaths then open your eyes. You should feel refreshed. It's common to fall asleep while meditating in Savasana, so don't worry if that happens to you. You may want to set an alarm before getting into the pose to make sure you don't sleep longer that you'd like.

Affirmations

We like the following affirmations to remind you how important you are:

· I am powerful.
· I am free to do what makes me happy.
· My opportunities are limitless.

Once again, choose your favorite way or ways to use affirmations and put them to work for you. We've summarized all the affirmations used in this book in Chapter 9. Feel free to refer to that chapter whenever you need a quick pick me up. We're sure you'll find the affirmation you need in that moment.

Meditation

A butterfly is commonly used as a symbol of transformation, and we've used it here in our book, because it represents one of the most dramatic transformations on earth. The almost slug-like caterpillar, stuck on the ground, wraps itself in its protective cocoon to emerge later as a beautiful butterfly with the ability to fly. Wow!

But a transformation journey is never truly over. As human beings, we are constantly growing and changing. We aren't meant to go through a transformation then stay at the place where we end up. Sure, some transformations will be more dramatic than others, but we will always be growing and changing.

For this last meditation, we thought it would be fun to honor the transformation process from caterpillar to butterfly. Find a comfortable spot and sit or lie down. Close your eyes and take a deep breath. Imagine you're a caterpillar crawling on a tree branch. You're looking for a good spot to make your cocoon. When you've found that spot, begin weaving your cocoon. You're surrounding yourself with layers and layers of comforting material, preparing to rest and let nature work its magic.

Once in your cocoon, breathe, sink into the darkness, and completely relax. When you feel it's time, feel your butterfly legs start to propel you out of your cocoon. Your wings are ready to expand and burst the confines of your cocoon. Feel how freeing it is to come out of your cocoon. You flap your wings, and soon you are soaring on the breeze. Open your wings, let all your fears go and just glide on the breeze for a moment.

When you're ready, embrace that feeling of freedom and hold it with you as you take three deep breaths, and open your eyes. You may want to take a moment and journal about your thoughts and feelings.

Of course, if a visualization doesn't feel right to you today, you can take some time to color or doodle. We also invite you to explore the extra coloring pages in Chapter 10.

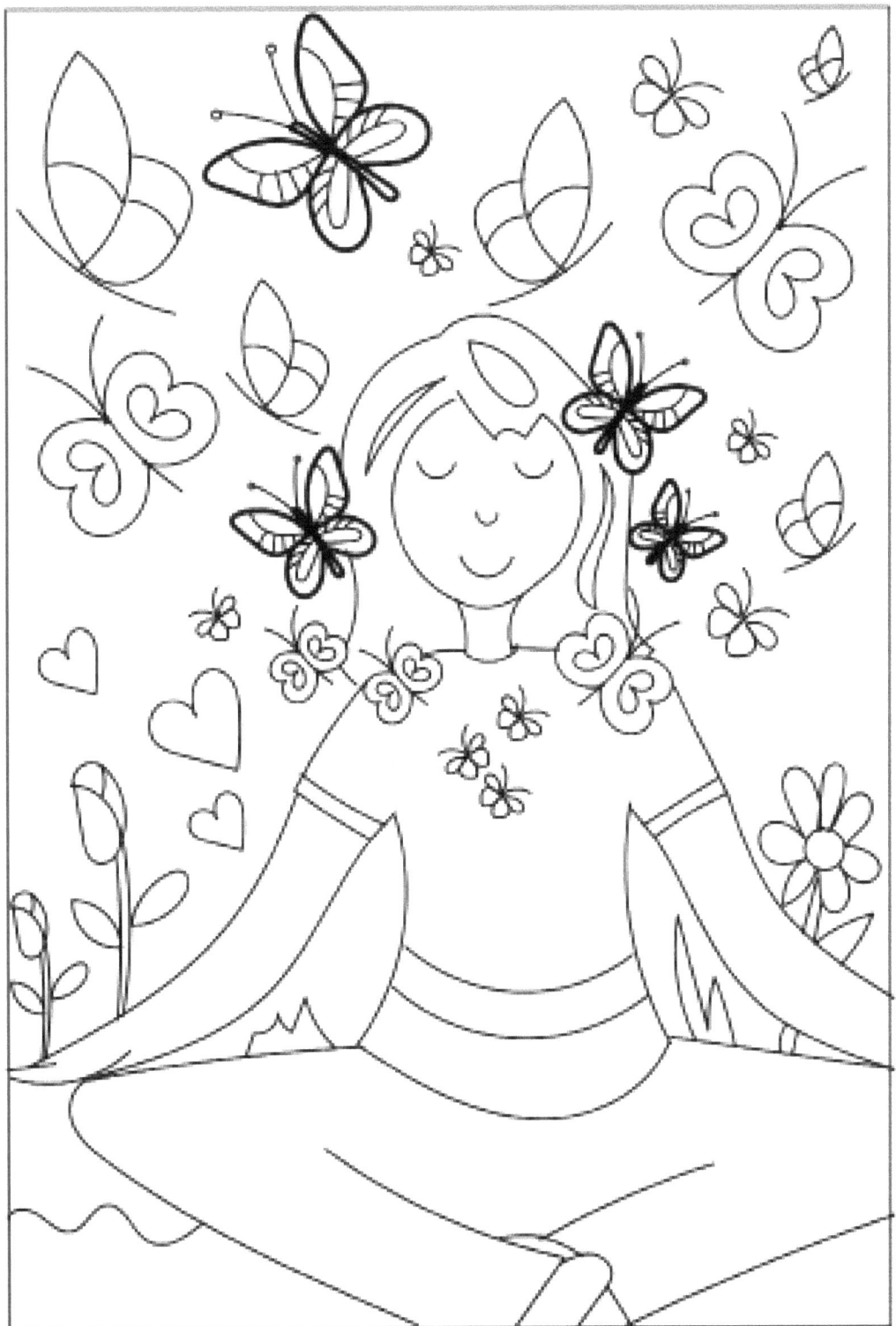

Use this page to **DOODLE**. If using markers, you may want to place extra paper or a piece of cardboard under this page to prevent bleed through. Have fun!

Crystals

We've mentioned several crystals throughout this book that are wonderful for working with the chakra system. Use the crystals you feel most drawn to, even if we haven't discussed them. There's a reason you are feeling drawn to working with them. As we close our discussion on crystals, we wanted to share with you some of our favorites and how we work with them.

Josie loves rose quartz and amethyst and her favorite way to use them is to place them on her body. Citrine and any variety of calcite are some of Michelle's favorites. She likes to use her crystals in whichever way she feels called to at the time. Some favorite ways are wearing them as jewelry, placing tiny stones in her bra, and placing quartz-based stones and calcite in the bath.

Remember, you don't need to buy a lot of crystals to benefit from them. You can use clear quartz for anything as long as you set your intention and ask the crystal to help you with whatever it is you need.

Essential Oils

As with the crystals, when working with your essential oils and the entire chakra system, we'd like you to choose the oils you feel most drawn to, the ones you have noticed the most benefits from, or the ones that ignite the happiest feelings. We'd like to share some of our favorite oils and how we use them.

Josie loves to diffuse chamomile and lavender oils. Michelle loves to diffuse her oils as well, but she also enjoys creating blends in carrier oils and rubbing them on her wrists. A favorite blend is equal amounts ylang ylang and frankincense in coconut oil.

If you've found an oil you really love, that's great. You don't need a whole lot of oils to benefit from them. Remember, lavender is a great oil to use with all the chakras.

Journal Prompt

We hope you've started journaling on a regular basis and our prompts have helped you examine what's preventing you from being the happiest version of yourself. We'd like to leave you with a releasing journal prompt you can use every day:

· What is preventing me from being happy today?

Write this at the top of your journal page and jot down anything that comes to mind. Remember to release any negative thoughts when you're done.

Every day is a new opportunity to learn something about ourselves. A gratitude journal prompt you can use every day is:

· I am grateful for learning _____ about myself today.

Fill in the blank with as many things that apply for that day.

Summary

You've come a long way and learned a lot about yourself in the process. Taking time for yourself has become a priority and you are becoming the happiest version of yourself. This quote from Nathaniel Hawthorne beautifully sums up the role taking time for yourself plays in your happiness:

"Happiness is a butterfly, which when pursued, is always just beyond your grasp, but which, if you will sit down quietly, may alight upon you."

Because a transformation is never truly over, and we want you to always feel like a free butterfly, we invite you to return to the pages of this book whenever you feel stuck.

Action Step

The action step for this chapter is simple: Remember to do something every day that makes you happy! Put it in your planner or phone if that helps you remember to make it a priority. Even the simplest things that bring a smile to your face count. Challenge yourself to do more and more happy things every day.

9

Affirming Your Happiness

Here are all the affirmations we've mentioned throughout the book listed by the stages represented in each chapter. A fun thing to do with this list is close your eyes then open them and see which affirmation they land on, and use that as your affirmation for the day. You can also close your eyes and use your finger to choose an affirmation or two. Wherever your finger is when you open your eyes, that's the affirmation you need to work with that day.

For recognizing your stuck (Chapter 1) . . .

· I feel safe and secure.
· I create my own happiness.
· I am ready to feel happy.

For committing to making a change (Chapter 2) . . .

· I have the power to change.
· I have what it takes to make a change.
· I can flourish.

For trying something new (Chapter 3) . . .

· I welcome new experiences.
· I find excitement in new experiences.
· I express myself in new ways.

For finding support (Chapter 4) . . .

· I am supported.
· I find support easily.
· I am connected.

For experimenting with new tools (Chapter 5) . . .

· I allow myself to try something different.
· I flow into happiness.
· I accept expansion every day.

For finding what works for you (Chapter 6) . . .

· I'm happy being me.
· I trust my intuition.
· I notice what makes me feel good.

For making time for yourself (Chapter 7) . . .

· I am stable, safe, and secure.
· I make time to care for myself.
· I am establishing a healthy routine.

For maintaining your freedom (Chapter 8) . . .

· I am powerful.
· I am free to do what makes me happy.
· My opportunities are limitless.

10

Coloring Your Happiest Life

"Color is a power which directly influences the soul."
—*Wassily Kandinsky*

We hope you've enjoyed the coloring pages as much as Michelle enjoyed creating them. As we mentioned in the introduction, coloring is a great activity for people who have a hard time quieting their mind during traditional meditation. The activities required to color (choosing colors and concentrating on staying inside the lines) give the brain something to focus on.

Besides promoting relaxation and reducing stress and anxiety, coloring also helps improve motor control and hand-eye coordination. Here are some bonus coloring pages for your enjoyment. Remember, if you like using markers, you'll want to put a piece of cardboard between your pages to prevent the markers from bleeding through to the next page.

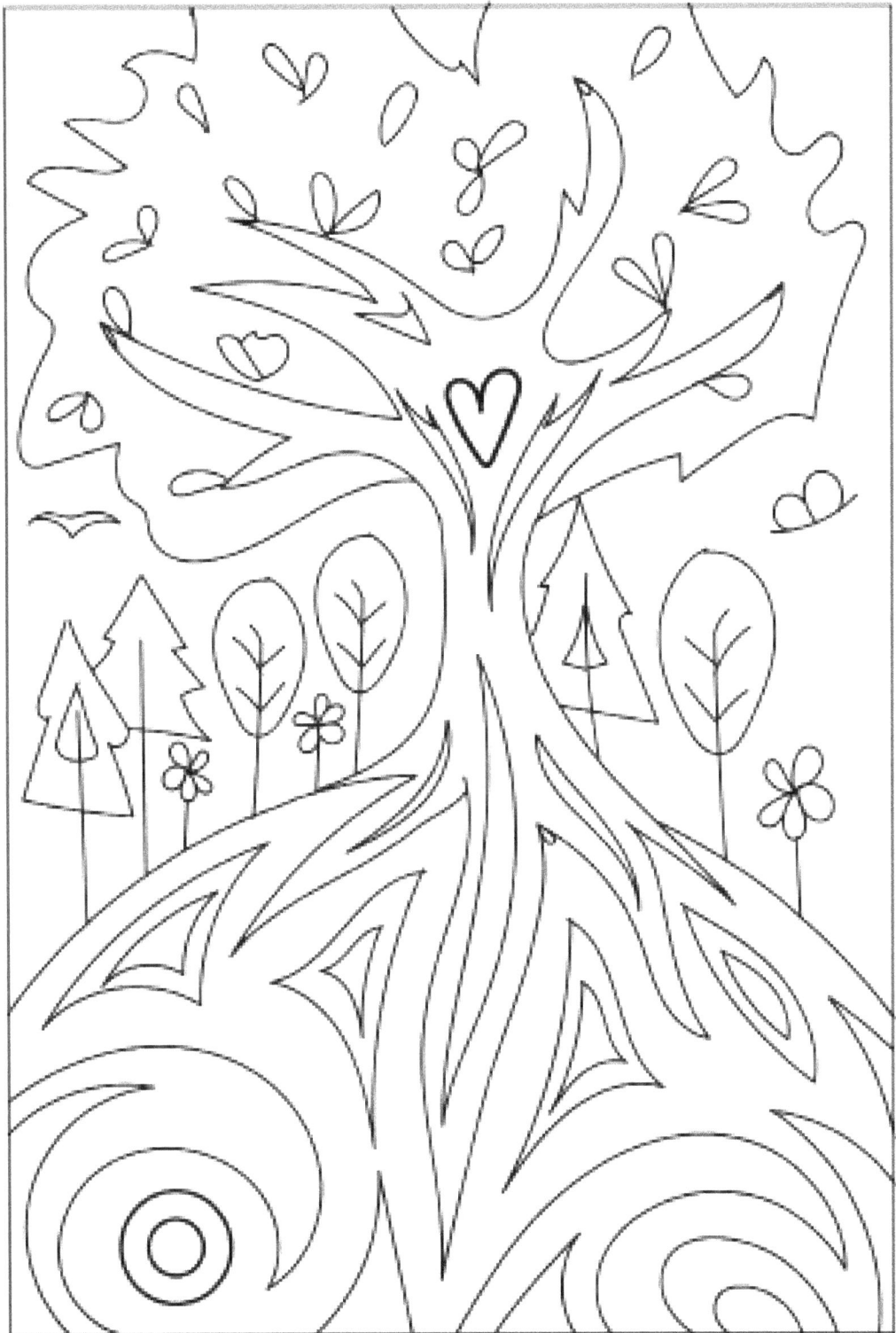

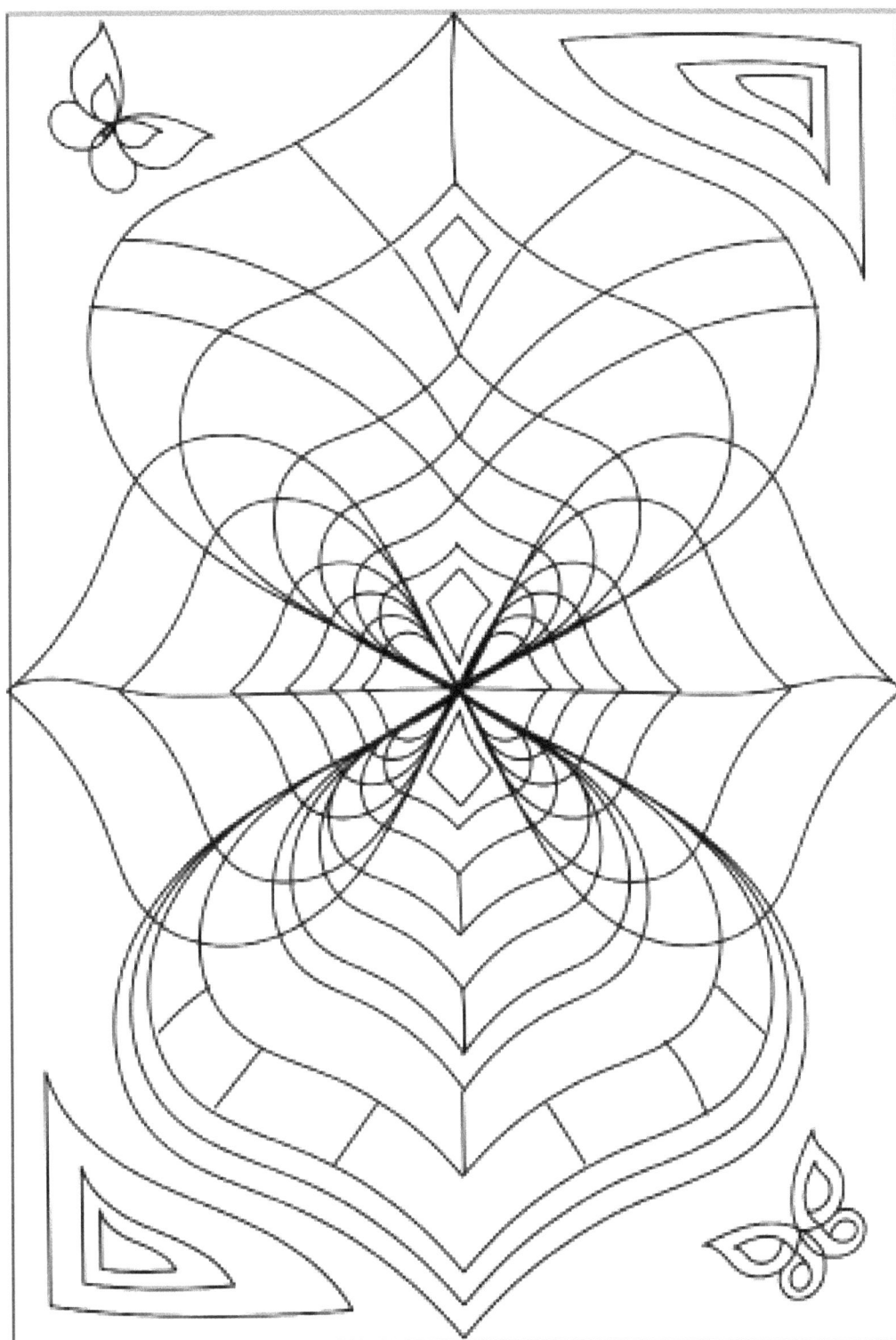

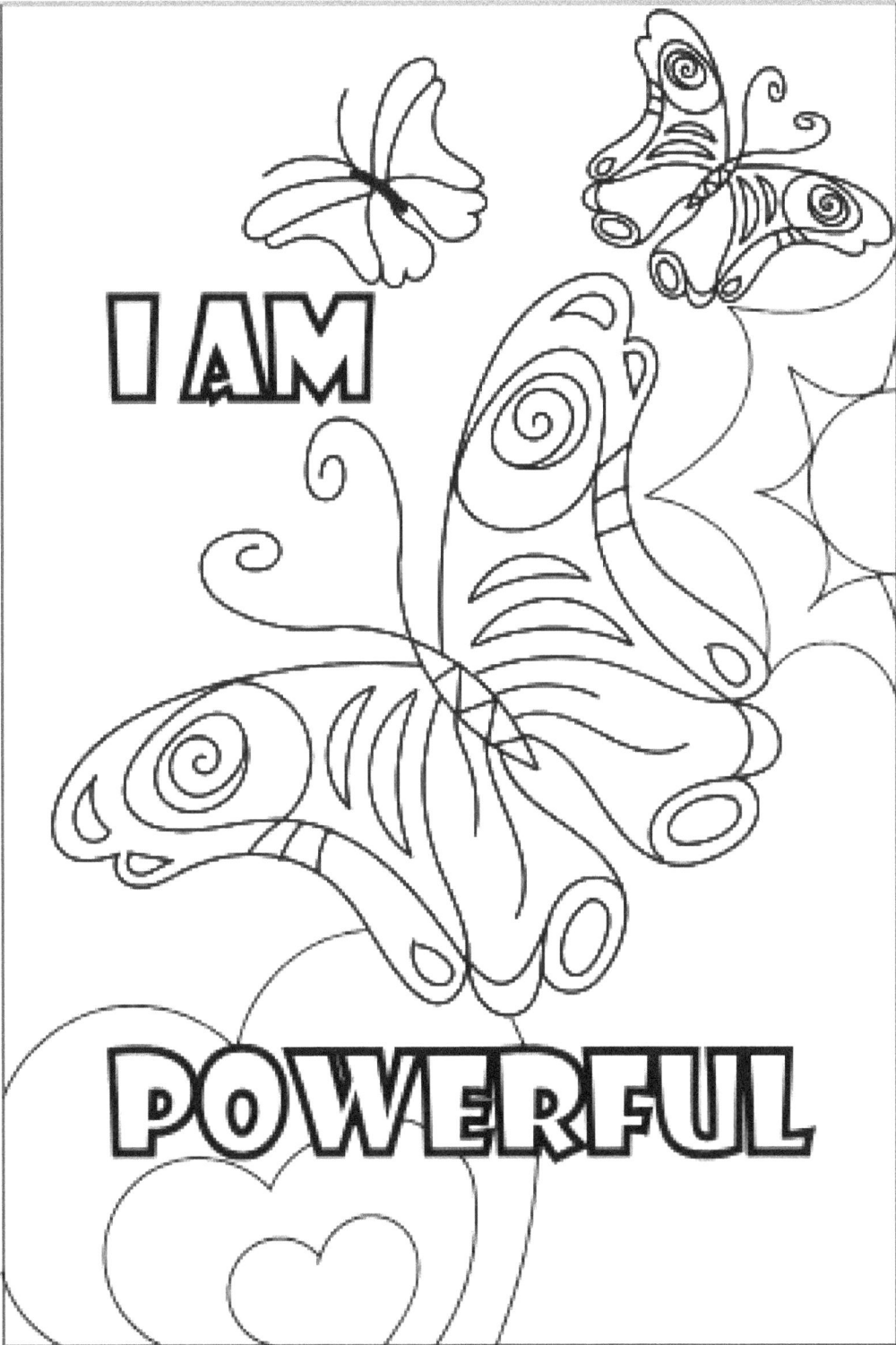

I AM

POWERFUL

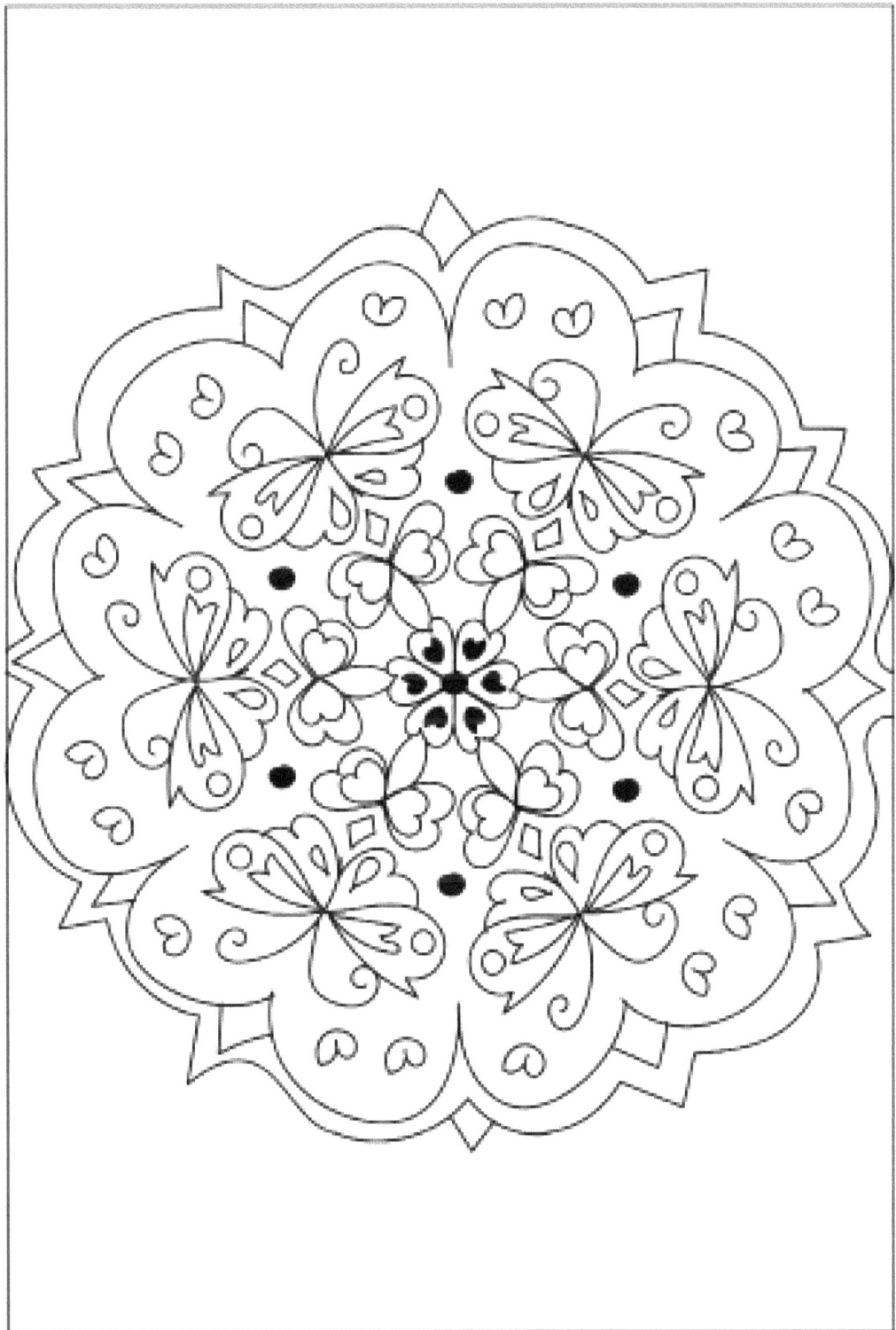

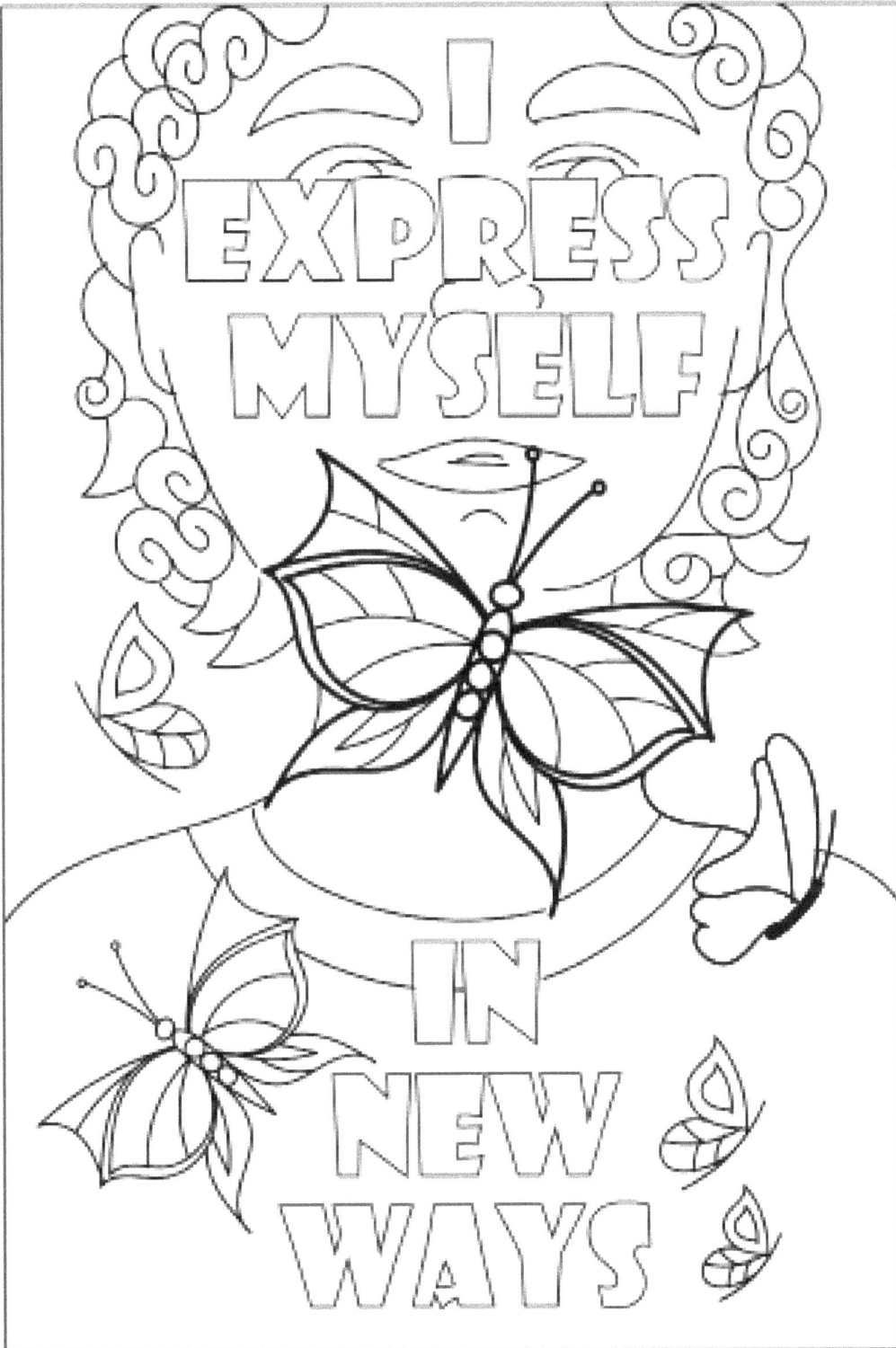

I EXPRESS MYSELF IN NEW WAYS

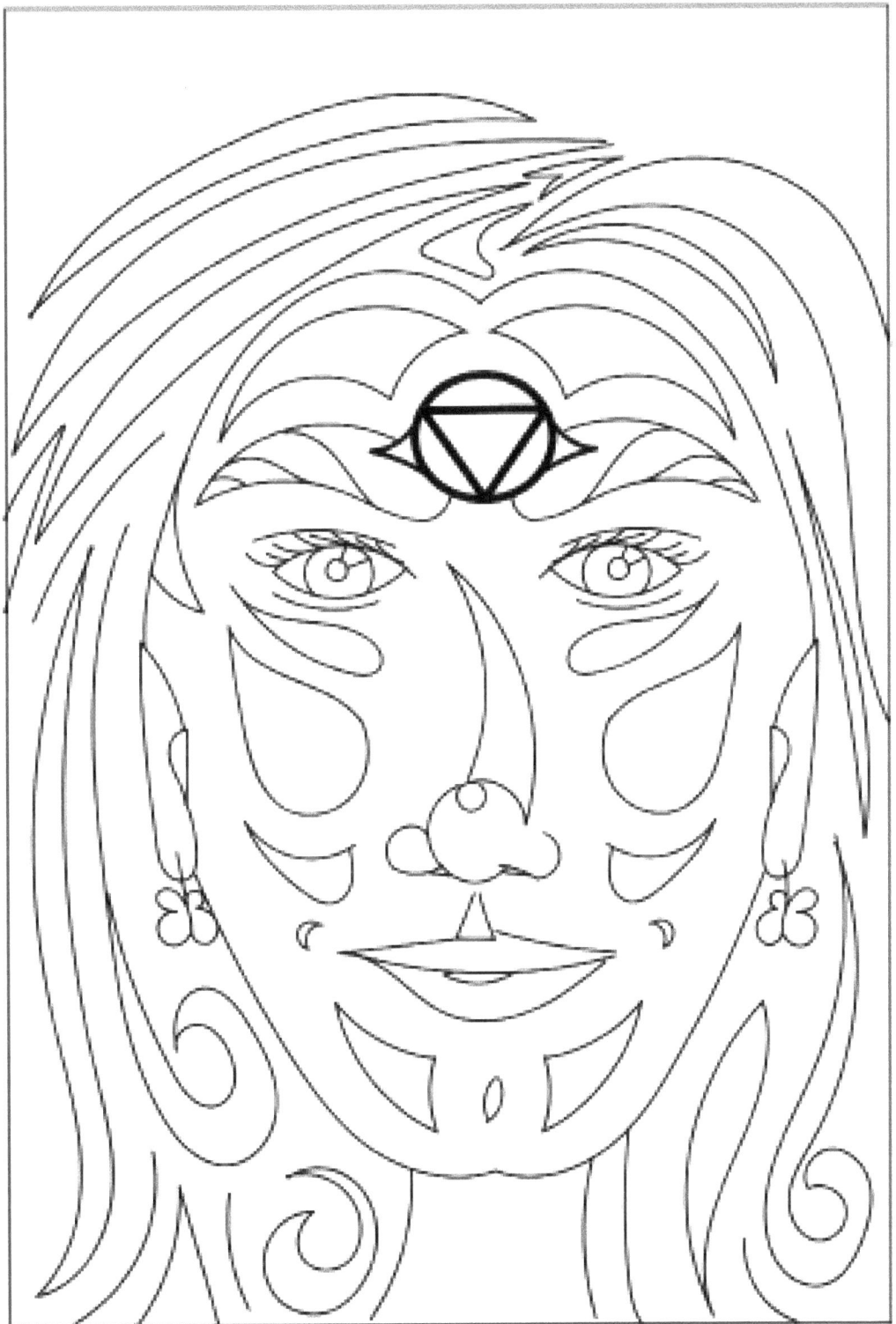

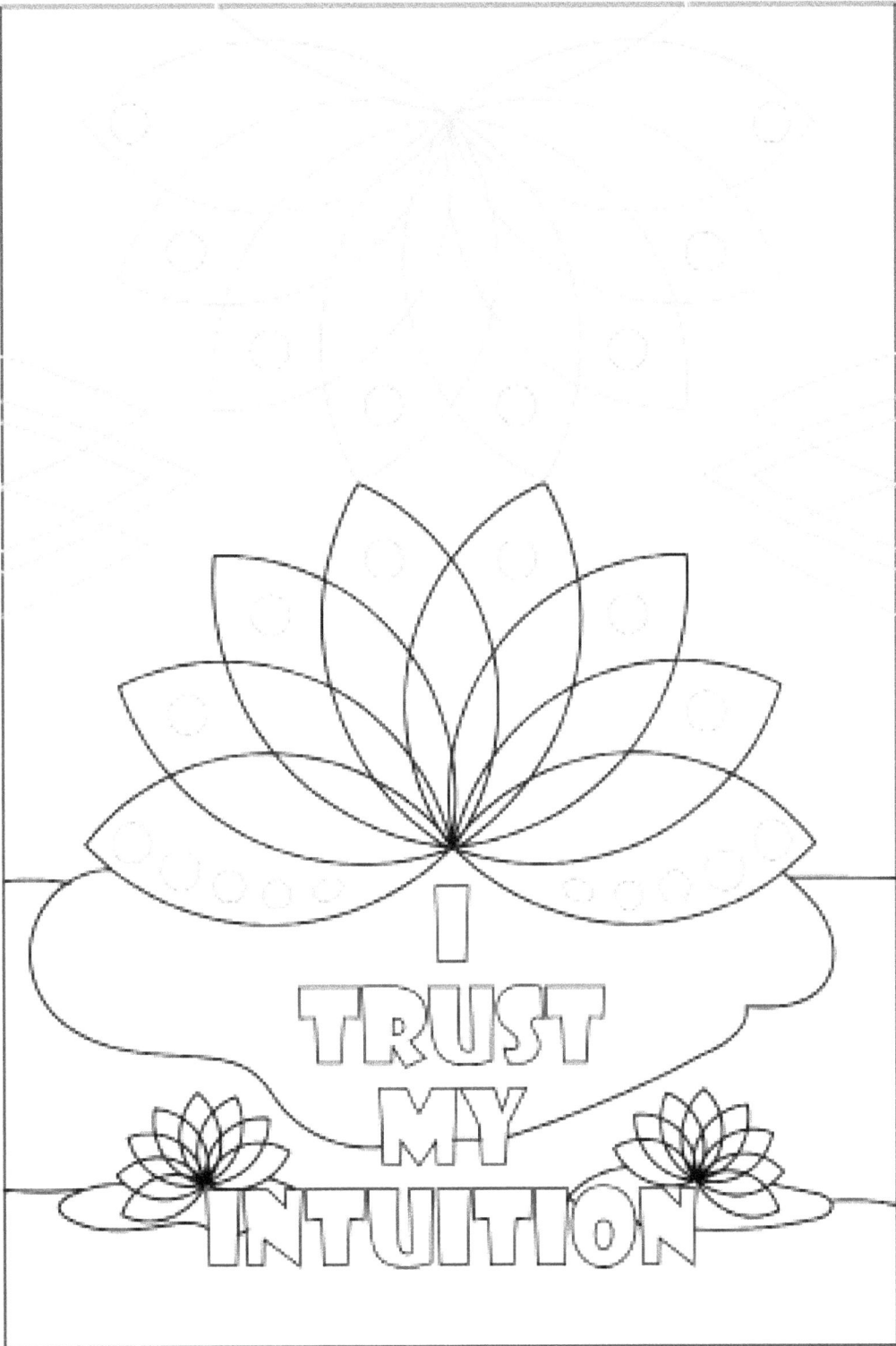

I
TRUST
MY
INTUITION

11

What if You're Still Stuck?

By Michelle

This past week, I got to look into a butterfly's eyes. They were fascinating and reminded me of tiny yellow marbles with faint lines painted over them that made what looked like an 'X'. And then I saw the eyes turn black when the butterfly died. My nine-year-old received a butterfly kit for his birthday. At this point there was one butterfly yet to emerge, two very lethargic butterflies, and one that had died with only its head poking out of its cocoon.

The excitement of teaching my kids about nature turned to wonder about the consequences of bringing nature indoors, of playing God with these little butterflies. If the butterfly had been raised in nature would it still have died?

Seeing the dead butterfly frozen half-way out of its cocoon got me thinking about our metaphor "freeing the butterfly". What happens when people are so stuck they can't move on? What if you've read this book, and you're still feeling stuck?

First of all, know that you aren't alone. I've been in this place myself, and know how it feels not to want to go on. There are anonymous hotlines and professionals that can help. Josie is an energy healer and Reiki Master offering in-person and online sessions. She has also felt the pain of wanting to end her own life. You can reach out to her here:

www.josiemyers.ca

There are also a number of organizations that can help. Here are a few to consider:

Crisis Services Canada: Canada Suicide Prevention Service

http://www.crisisservicescanada.ca/
1-833-456-4566

Suicide Prevention Lifeline

https://suicidepreventionlifeline.org/
1-800-273-8255

The International Bipolar Foundation provides a list of suicide hotlines by country. We have reprinted this list from their website (https://ibpf.org/resource/list-international-suicide-hotlines).

Argentina: +5402234930430

Australia: 131114

Austria: 017133374

Belgium: 106

Bosnia & Herzegovina: 080 05 03 05

Botswana: 3911270

Brazil: 188 for the CVV National Association

Canada: 514 723 4000 (Montreal); 1 866 277 3553 (outside Montreal)

Croatia: 014833888

Denmark: +4570201201

Egypt: 7621602

Estonia: 3726558088; in Russian 3726555688

Finland: 010 195 202

France: 0145394000

Germany: 08001810771

Holland: 09000767

Hong Kong: +852 2382 0000

Hungary: 116123

India: 8888817666

Ireland: +4408457909090

Italy: 800860022

Japan: +810352869090

Mexico: 5255102550

New Zealand: 0800543354

Norway: +4781533300

Philippines: 028969191

Poland: 5270000

Portugal: 21 854 07 40/8 . 96 898 21 50

Russia: 0078202577577

Spain: 914590050

South Africa: 0514445691

Sweden: 46317112400

Switzerland: 143

United Kingdom: 08457909090

USA: 1 800 273 8255

Veterans' Crisis Line: 1 800 273 8255/ text 838255

References & Recommended Reading

Horsley, Mary. 2007. *Chakra Workout: Balancing Your Energy with Yoga and Meditation*, Sterling, New York, NY.

Loomis, K. Kris. 2016. *How to Sneak More Meditation Into Your Life: A Doable Meditation Plan for Busy People*. Lililoom Publishing, Rock Hill, SC.

Loomis, K. Kris. 2016. *How to Sneak More Yoga Into Your Life: A Doable Yoga Plan for Busy People*. Lililoom Publishing, Rock Hill, SC.

Northrup, Christiane. 2016. *Goddesses Never Age: The Secret Prescription for Radiance, Vitality, and Well-Being.* Hay House Inc., Carlsbad, CA.

Perrakis, Athena. 2018. *The Ultimate Guide to Chakras: The Beginner's Guide to Balancing, Healing, and Unblocking Your Chakras for Health and Positive Energy.* Fair Winds Press, Beverly, MA.

Perrakis, Athena. 2019. *Crystal Lore, Legends, and Myth: The Fascinating History of the World's Most Powerful Gems and Stones.* Fair Winds Press, Beverly, MA.

Subject Index

www.ingramcontent.com/pod-product-compliance
Lightning Source LLC
Chambersburg PA
CBHW042349030426
42336CB00025B/3426